D0149729

FREEING THE BODY
FREEING THE MIND

FREEING THE BODY FREEING THE MIND

WRITINGS ON THE CONNECTIONS BETWEEN YOGA AND BUDDHISM

EDITED BY

MICHAEL STONE

foreword by

ROBERT THURMAN

SHAMBHALA

BOSTON & LONDON 2010

Shambhala Publications, Inc.
Horticultural Hall
300 Massachusetts Avenue
Boston, Massachusetts 02115
www.shambhala.com

9 8 7 6 5 4 3 2

Printed in the United States of America

♾ This edition is printed on acid-free paper that meets the American National Standards Institute z39.48 Standard.
♻ This book was printed on 30% postconsumer recycled paper. For more information please visit www.shambhala.com.

Distributed in the United States by Random House, Inc., and in Canada by Random House of Canada Ltd

Designed by Dede Cummings Designs

Library of Congress Cataloging-in-Publication Data

Freeing the body, freeing the mind: writings on the connections between yoga and Buddhism / edited by Michael Stone; foreword by Robert Thurman.—1st ed.

p. cm.

Includes bibliographical references.

ISBN 978-1-59030-801-1 (pbk.: alk. paper)

1. Yoga—Buddhism. I. Stone, Michael, 1974–

BQ4610.Y63F74 2010

294.3'4436—dc22

2010006462

CONTENTS

FOREWORD

THE WONDERFUL THING about writing a foreword for a good book is having to read the book through first. American life tends toward busyness, and often we are compelled to put down without finishing even an excellent book that serves to reveal more of reality to our awareness. But on duty with this book, I read every word with delight. I contemplated each exercise, I appreciated the many insights, and I was moved by the stories of the contributors. Adapting the felicitous phrase of Thich Nhat Hanh, I "inter-read," and enjoyed "inter-being" with the realm of the book.

Furthermore, since the topic is Yoga and Buddhism, reading the accounts of these accomplished teachers, dipping into their stories, sharing their streams of experiences and insights—and their valuable and eloquently presented teachings—is like having a bit of a retreat. Calmness, awareness, wisdom, kindness, and compassion bubble up in the pages of this book and make it a joy to visit. Those deep into Buddhism can find a lot to help their understanding and meditation practice in the wisdom and embodying practicality of the Yoga tradition. Those deep into Yoga can find enriching dimensions in the Buddhist Yogas presented herein. And the broad range of readers can find practical help, methods, and tools for a better health, life, and state of mind in the integrated paths presented.

I have always maintained that Buddhism can make its best contribution to our modern culture by offering its multifarious methods and insights without insisting on being Buddhism, and certainly Yoga is in essence a highly skillful way of being realistic about the body. The essays here encourage taking responsibility for one's own health, cultivating a stronger sense of meaning in one's life, finding the inner strength to express joyful altruism, and developing an artful connoisseurship toward enjoying every moment as if it is the ultimate in every sense.

I especially enjoy the sincerity and depth of Michael Stone and the writers he has invited to contribute to this feast of insights. During the fifty years I have been learning, studying, practicing, teaching, and trying to perform the Buddhist teachings, there were long decades when it seemed that American people were intently preoccupied with the pursuit of money, status, possessions, and experiences of pleasure, and unrelentingly unconscious of the impact of their lifestyle on the world around them.

In academia, one doesn't really teach the Dharma; one can only teach *about* the Dharma, the history of Buddhism, Hinduism, Jainism, Indian civilization, the philosophies of the great masters, the literatures produced, and so on. Young people are launched into the world as graduates with lots of skills and information, and with some adeptness in critical analysis for scientific wisdom—but absolutely no training in how to use the mind's higher faculties through cultivation of mindfulness, one-pointed concentration, and wisdom's critical insight meditation. Even ethical awareness is only developed haphazardly through immersion in literary classics or the occasional philosophical study of various ethical systems. And what has been appropriately called "emotional intelligence," the self-knowledge of the workings of emotional and conceptual conditioning and reactivity that is essential to a person's living of a good life, is absolutely ignored.

Therefore, books such as this are essential to the continuing curriculum of hopefully ever greater numbers of students in order for them really to be prepared to live a meaningful, productive, altruistic, and satisfying life, and make a positive contribution to our globalizing society.

I welcome it, I heartily congratulate the editor and the contributors, I salute the publishers, and I strongly recommend it to readers of all ages, and all walks of life.

Robert Tenzin Thurman
Jey Tsong Khapa Professor of
Indo-Tibetan Buddhist Studies,
Columbia University
President, Tibet House, U.S.

TIMELINE

THIS TIMELINE OFFERS approximate dates of authors, teachers, and texts referred to throughout this collection.

2000 C.E.	1888–1989	Krishnamacharya
	1863–1902	Swami Vivekananda
	17th–18th c.	Śiva Samhita
	17th c.	Gerandha-Samhitā
	15th–16th c.	Svātmārāma
1500 C.E.	15th c.	Haṭha Yoga Pradīpikā
	1200–1253	Dōgen
	1100–1200	Yoga Vaśiṣṭa
1000 C.E.	1000	Goraksha birth of Hatha Yoga
	788–820	Śaṅkarācārya
	8th c.	birth of Kashmir Shaivism
	8th c.	Padmasambhava
	600	Heart Sūtra
	6th–7th c.	Vajrayāna
500 C.E.	5th c.	Bodhidharma
	150	Patañjali
	150–250	Nagarjuna
	2nd c.	Sāṃkhya Karika of Īśvarakrsna
C.E.		
B.C.E		
500 B.C.E.		
	563–483	Gautama Buddha
	600	Bhagavad Gītā
	800–100	Upaniṣads
1000 B.C.E.		
1500 B.C.E.		
	1700–1100	Ṛg Veda

INTRODUCTION

THIS BOOK IS written for those who, like myself, find themselves not only compelled by the teachings and practices of both Yoga and Buddhism, but also moved to better understand the porous border between them. Whether described in terms of transcendence, enlightenment, freedom, compassion, or deep stages of meditative quietude, both Yoga and the Dharma taught by the Buddha and his disciples have a long interdependent history weaving backward from present-day Western culture through Tibet, India, Mongolia, China, Japan, Thailand, Korea, Burma, and many other countries. These various strands of practice all share the unifying goal of recognizing suffering and bringing it to an end.

The Buddha was not only exposed to diverse Yoga practices, he was himself a yogi who wandered from the known cultural milieu of his time into the dense forests and open deltas of the Ganges seeking to bring an end to his relentless existential questions. Looking into the entanglements of his mind and the flux of reality as it manifested in his body, the Buddha made a pilgrimage in the external sense—leaving cultural and familial comforts for the unpopulated natural world; and also internally—settling his breath, mind, and body into one another until a clear and quiet awareness appeared under the surface distractions of consciousness. On discovering the innate stability of awareness, he found true freedom in the body and mind—a freedom that revealed the truth that nothing moving through awareness refers back to a central or locatable self.

For too long, Western interpretations of Yoga and Buddhism have separated one from the other by narrowly describing Yoga as a body practice while characterizing the Dharma teachings of the Buddha as exclusively mind practices. Such oversimplification not only misrepresents the two traditions but also disregards the long history of dialogue that both Yoga and Buddhism share and the complex ethical, philosophical, and cultural components that underscore each system.

If we imagine the traditions of Yoga and Buddhism as two trees, perhaps an oak and a maple, at first these two systems seem quite similar: we can characterize them as being trees, relying on water and photosynthesis, containing multitudes of leaves and branches and roots that extend deep into the earth. But as any simple observation reveals, maple trees and oak trees are quite different from each other; they require different amounts of water, they grow branches in quite dissimilar patterns, and the leaves of the oak, with their fine detail, hardly resemble those of the maple. If I were painting an oak leaf and a maple leaf, I'd use a different palette of colors for each; the lines that represent their internal structure would bear little resemblance; and if I tried to capture the way their leaves change color and decay in autumn, I'd have to sit under the maple well in advance of the oak. Yet, if I were to continue this observation one step further, the similarities between the two trees would start to become clear once again: their roots systems grow in congruent ways, and their respective leaf patterns and growth cycles follow the seasons in very similar ways. When comparing two systems, whether trees or complex spiritual traditions, when we look for parallel comparisons, we find difference, and when we look for difference, we find similarity.

Yoga and Buddhism are as complex as the ecology of trees, and like trees they share characteristic patterns that reveal some profound similarities—similarities that in turn teach us about ourselves, the way we construct the world, our attempts to deal with suffering and anguish, and the human possibility of cultivating genuine altruistic action. Both traditions draw on mind and body practices, ethical contemplation and action, a turning inward of attention in order to still psychophysical distractions, and a path to awakening. Are the paths of Yoga and Buddhism truly separate? Are they pointing at similar truths or are they speaking about different categories of awakening? Obviously a book of this size cannot adequately deal with the variations, differences, and combinations of all the various schools within what we call "Yoga" and "Buddhism," but can help us understand what these two traditions are asking of those who undertake committed practice.

While the themes of the contributors are varied, the main thrust of this book has to do with the possibility of freedom and how great teachers like the Buddha, Patañjali, Dōgen, and Nagarjuna, among others, understood freedom and consequently described a path, or at least reputable techniques, that create the conditions for genuine realization. All of the contributors herein are practitioners first and thinkers second, and we are all writing from personal experience having practiced within and between these two systems for many years. Although the situation is slowly changing, there is still a significant disparity between academics and practitioners, and the English literature on Yoga practice suffers from this more than the Buddhist. Looking at traditions like Yoga and Buddhism as mere philosophies, especially without practicing the techniques described within them, is not good science, good research, or good history. A purely intellectual approach to these practices leaves the core teachings unexamined, and in such cases the scholar is blinded by his or her books. Therefore, this book attempts to describe not only the philosophical basis of Yoga and Buddhism but also what it's like to practice within and between these systems.

If we take the Buddha and Patañjali as leading figures of the two traditions we are comparing, it's perhaps unsettling to learn that we know very little of the personal history of either of them. We know Patañjali only through his short aphorisms and attributed mythology, and we know the Buddha primarily through the early writings of the Pali canon, which began being compiled over a century after his death. About the Buddha, Karen Armstrong writes:

> After his enlightenment we get no sense of his likes and dislikes, his hopes and fears, moments of desperation, elation, or intense striving. What remains is an impression of a transhuman serenity, self-control, a nobility that has gone beyond the superficiality of

> personal preference, and a profound equanimity. The Buddha is often compared to non-human beings—to animal, trees, or plants—not because he is subhuman or inhumane, but because he has utterly transcended the selfishness that most of us regard as inseparable from our condition.[1]

Gautama Buddha, like other leading figures in the Yoga tradition, clarified for us what it means to be human and what liberation from lack and suffering (duḥkha) might look like. But we can only know such awakening for ourselves. Furthermore, if we can know awakening only through this subjective life—through our particular mind-body process—the only place we can begin a reasonable investigation into reality is here and now in *this* mind, in *this* body. It's not just distractedness and habitual preferences that we come up against in our attempt to see through the illusions and constructs that veil the mind's clarity and the heart's potential for compassion, it's self-centeredness. Karen Armstrong continues her description of the Buddha:

> In the West, we prize individualism and self-expression, but this can easily degenerate into mere self-promotion. What we find in Gautama is a complete and breathtaking self-abandonment. He would have been surprised to learn that the scriptures do not present him as a fairly rounded "personality," but would have said that our concept of personality was a dangerous delusion.[2]

Our discontent and delusions stem from the ways we create a false and separate self that, over time, feels like a subject in relation to a body. Since we no longer live in a sense-absorbed natural environment in which we are constantly attending to the feel of the wind or the changing weather patterns, and since we live primarily indoors, we have come to rely on the mental sphere much more than the other sense media. This comes at a price. Our attention span is so short and easily interrupted that we no longer have the sensitivity to the other senses that we would have if we lived outdoors. We don't need to navigate the physical world in the same way we once did, so as modern people we are relying too much on the mind's proliferation at the expense of the other senses.

Even in Buddha's time, the body was used as the primary object of meditation so that one could study the universe not through books or theory but through one's subjective experience. Likewise the Yoga postures, when practiced with breathing and sensitivity, become opportunities for deep meditative insight because they are designed to calm the nervous system and return us to earth. When we tune in to the internal energetic patterns of the breath as we move within the various shapes of the Yoga poses, we are, in essence, working the habits of the mind as well. Though the Yoga postures we practice in modern Yoga studios have obvious therapeutic benefits at physiological levels, we seem to have forgotten how the postures also teach us how to work with the mind. And for most of us, our troubles are not simply in the body but primarily in the mind. How can we use the body to study the mind and work with the mind through the body? We do so by seeing and experiencing how the two are completely interrelated.

There is a fundamental affinity between mind practices and body practices because they are both simply curves in a grand concentric circle that continually spirals in, on, and through itself with no beginning or end. Work deeply with the mind and you give attention to body processes from breathing to listening or seeing. Likewise, when you study the intricate holding patterns in the web of the body (called kośas in Sanskrit), you end up seeing where the mind sticks, where it can't focus, where it gets caught in refrains of old tape loops. What you thought was "body" is mostly mental, not "the body in the body" that the Buddha says to direct mindfulness toward. When the Buddha teaches mindfulness practices, he begins with the body.

Each of the many schools within Yoga and Buddhist traditions may touch universal truths about human experience and the transformation of suffering, yet it's important to remember that each school arises out of particular cultural conditions. Indian Hatha Yoga and Tibetan tantric practices have many similarities and roots, but the way they are described and performed are influenced by the cultures in which they've been refined. The metaphoric language and esoteric maps of the tantric traditions (Tibet) bear little resemblance to the dry psychology of Buddhist Abhidharma (India) or the ferocious clarity of Nagarjuna's deconstruction of language (Tibet). Even the Buddha's teachings changed depending on what and to whom he was teaching. As Hatha Yoga practices become increasingly popular in North America, Europe, and Asia, we also see very unique characteristics in the emerging culture of Yoga, among which are commercial Yoga studios, teacher training programs, and a new focus on the physical and muscular geometry of Yoga postures with perhaps less attention to the subtle winds of the breath, ethics, or the stillness of sitting practice.

Buddhism also looks different in the West than it does in Japan, China, and Burma, with less of a monastic population, many more lay practitioners, and a strong focus on meditation practice. As both Yoga and Buddhism enter into dialogue with each other, as they each plant seeds in modern secular culture, it's important that we understand these traditions as shifting descriptions of reality and not fixed truths untouched by cultural traditions. As soon as we call something a "system," we narrow it down within specific cultural parameters, and unfortunately if we focus too much on the form of the system, we might forget what it's pointing at. No system is created or practiced in a vacuum. The *Upaniṣads* were a response and refinement of the *Vedas,* and early Buddhism another radical refinement of Upaniṣadic wisdom.

The Buddha moved beyond the notion of freedom as something one finds somewhere else. Liberation for the Buddha did not come by touching something inside oneself, through finding something in the beyond, or by having faith in a creator-god, but rather through the process of waking up to *this* ground; not waking up to the fixed nature of reality but waking up to the way things happen. This process reveals the groundless ground of transience, the temporary nature of how things come into being and then pass away again—not the eternal notion of a savior beyond space and time.

The sages, seers, and yogis of ancient India or the poet-artist-students of medieval Japan did not develop their practices in idyllic conditions of peace and quietude. "And if you are born into a heavenly realm of peace and stillness," one of my teachers once said to me, "it's bad for your Yoga practice because there is not enough suffering to motivate you to practice." Even in the European and American Yoga "scene" we can begin to see a more wholistic approach to Hatha Yoga emerging in which students are beginning to expand their practice beyond the physical practice to include sitting meditation, prāṇāyāma, chanting, and textual study. Eventually, perhaps, these commercial Yoga studios may even become community centers where Yoga is offered and taught to the diverse members of the community including the aged, the ill, and families.

Yoga shows up in times of distress, when the principal paradigms and religious practices don't offer enough of a solution to our internal discord. Sometimes the dominant cultural institutions can't offer us the answers we hope will put an end to our suffering, so we must leave behind the answers being offered all around us and instead turn to the basic questions that being born and having to die press upon each and every one of us. Being separated from those we love, living in bodies that are aging and prone to illness, and discovering that we are not being skillful in working with habitual energies of the mind and emotions, motivate us to slow down and pay attention to the basic truths of being alive. When we look to the causes of violence and hatred, even in contemporary times, we do not have to look far; for if we look into our own psyche, our own body, our own families and communities, we can begin to see the psychological causes at work. The yogis of old have continually turned to their own minds and bodies, to the breath and the natural world, as sources of inspiration for awakening, and not to the "ready" answers that the dominant culture promotes. We see our holding patterns appear in our own bodies, our intimate relationships, and the habitual grooves of our minds.

"The old Indian practice of Yoga," writes scholar Karen Armstrong, "meant that people became dissatisfied with a religion that concentrated on externals. Sacrifice and liturgy were not enough: they wanted to discover the inner meaning of these rites."[3] Turning inward means taking responsibility for the spiritual path by focusing on the microcosm of reality that exists in the body's functioning in this and every moment. Although yogic practices can supposedly be traced back some five thousand years, and although yogins described their paths and discoveries in very different terms depending on their respective cultural vocabulary, they share the same common focus: the body as the primary object of meditative inquiry. When we begin by taking care of the body and paying attention to its workings, we find ourselves focusing the mind, settling the breath, and learning much more about the nature of reality than we'd know by extraverted thinking alone. There are some things we just can't figure out with ordinary thinking.

Chip Hartranft and Frank Jude Boccio both explore the way their own Buddhist and Yogic practices interweave, and they set their respective practices against the backdrop of traditional teachings. Though Roshi Pat Enkyo O'Hara does not refer to her own Yoga practice, she draws deeply on her Zen insight to explore the way we can touch our most basic and creative self through the dropping away of our self-concepts. Mu Soeng, codirector of the Barre Center for Buddhist Studies, has written a controversial and important chapter on the way both Yoga and Buddhist practices can slip into mechanical and unconscious patterns for which we must be vigilant. Daniel Odier and Eido Shimano Roshi have explored the body from the perspectives of Zen and Ch'an respectively and in so doing help break down the false view that meditation is a mind practice divorced from the body and the sensuality of the breath. Victoria Austin articulates her unique perspective as both a Zen teacher and an Iyengar Yoga teacher and in so doing draws some fascinating parallels between what a new student to each tradition might experience in their first foray into practice, including some of the similarities and differences of Yoga and Zen. Ari Goldfield, a stellar translator of Tibetan Buddhism, and his partner Rose Taylor, a longtime Buddhist and Yoga practitioner, draw on the Tibetan understanding of the term of *Yoga* along with the tantric practices that underpin a mature understanding of the nature of body and mind in Tibetan Buddhism. Christopher Chapple, one of the most prominent scholars of Yoga in the United States and also a longtime practitioner, draws some fascinating parallels between traditional Yoga and Buddhist teachings. In so doing he paves the way for future conversations about the way in which these systems have continually drawn from each other in the course of their maturation and how as contemporary practitioners we cannot easily divorce one system from another. Jill Satterfield tells the story of how Yoga and Buddhism have been integrated not just in her teaching but also in a dramatic transformation in her own body and heart. Lastly, Sarah Powers has brought together her unique synthesis of Hatha Yoga, yin practices, and Buddhist training, and has offered a very personal and accessible account of what it's like to practice both Yoga and the Buddhadharma day in and day out.

By "the body," these ancient traditions are not referring to the body in relation to the world: large, small, healthy, beautiful, round—but rather to the sense of the body as a frame of reference. Just resting in feeling the sense of the body without any notions or concepts, we begin to tune in to the glorious operation of the natural world only available to a quiet mind. Of course, the mind is not separate from the body in any way, just a seamless continuation of the sense organs. We begin with the body because it is always present, always grounded, and the very apparatus we need to receive and explore any corner of the natural world. We use "the mind" to explore "the body," but as we get closer and quieter, we come to see that mind and body are inseparable. The seeker Uddālaka in the *Yoga Vaśiṣṭa,* a story that interweaves Yoga and Buddhist philosophy, enters a remote practice place and begins practicing Yoga. After some time he exclaims,

> Just as the silkworm spins its cocoon and gets caught in it, you have woven the web of your concepts and are caught in them.
>
> . . . There is no such thing as mind. I have carefully investigated, I have observed everything from the tips of my toes to the top

of my head: and I have not found anything of which I could say: This is who I am.[4]

If we approach Yoga practices simply through books and words, and not direct contact with the physical and material reality of the body and breath, all we are left with is conceptual scaffolding. We can't know these practices from the outside; they were never meant to be mere philosophy or codified ritual. Knowing *about* practice is not enough, for we must drop our "knowing" and feel our way into present experience by seeing things clearly. By seeing, the old yogis are not referring to the eyes but to what the Zen tradition calls "the true dharma eye"—the eye that sees without clinging, without sculpting, without allowing what is seen to get stuck in this or that, like or dislike. The spirit of Yoga and Buddhism embodies a radical approach to human experience whereby we begin practice through paying attention to what is here in this moment, allowing each and every one of us to wake up without needing to adopt a new ideology or belief system. When we return to present experience through the sense organs themselves—eyes, ears, nose, tongue, skin, and mind—we enter the freedom of this very moment, and the old paths of the yogis come alive here and now. There is no freedom in just repeating the words and rituals of the old masters—we must express freedom and interdependence through the actions of our whole being, and community, through mind, body, and speech.

Every morning we wake up under the same bright northern star the Buddha saw when he awoke one dawn in his early thirties. Every moment we breathe the same molecules of air that once nourished Śāntideva, Dōgen, Thich Nhat Hanh, your parents, and their parents. Perhaps practice fulfills a responsibility to the yogi-poets and wanderers that long ago traveled the great magnificent rivers of this human body and then took great care in putting together words and phrases as they tried to leave helpful maps we can now pick up, compare, and put to use.

May this book help clarify your practice.

SANSKRIT PRONUNCIATION

IN THIS COLLECTION there are Tibetan, Japanese, Pali, and Sanskrit terms. Because Sanskrit is the dominant technical vocabulary used throughout the collection, I've offered diacritical marks throughout the text to help you familiarize yourself with these common yogic/Buddhist terms. The following is a guide to pronouncing Sanskrit terms:

There are five Sanskrit diacritic markings in the text:

A line above the letter (ā)

A dot above the letter (ṅ)

A dot below the letter (ḍ)

A tilde above the letter (ñ)

An acute accent above the letter (ś)

a (short) is like the *a* in *sofa,* as in the word *manas* (mind).

ā (long) is like the *a* in *father,* as in *āsana.*

i (short) is like the *i* in *pin*, as in *cit.*

ī (long) is like the *i* in *pique,* as in *jīva* (soul).

u (short) is like the *u* in *put,* as in *guṇa.*

ū (long) is like the *u* in *rule,* as in *rūpa* (form).

ṛ is pronounced like the *ri* in *rivet* and is usually found in *Kṛṣṇa.*

au is like the *o* in *how,* as in *Gautama Buddha.*

c is like the *ch* in *church* and never pronounced like *k* in *car* or *s* in *sent.* An example of this is *cakra* or *cit.*

ñ is palatal and nasal, like the *ny* in *canyon* or the word *onion,* and this is how a name like *Patañjali* is pronounced.

ṣ or ś are pronounced as *sh,* though the tongue position of ś is palatal and the tongue position of *ṣ* has the tip of the tongue at the roof of the mouth, as found in the English *shun* and the romanized Sanskrit word *Śūnyata.*

Although Sanskrit words are not pluralized by adding an *s* the way English words are, we've used the *s* in such terms as *āsanas,* in order to ease readability in English. Any errors in the diacritical marks and spelling of Sanskrit terms are mine; I added the diacritical marks after the authors signed off on their chapters.

1

AWAKENING TO PRĀṆA

CHIP HARTRANFT

SURVEYING THE CONTEMPORARY landscape of Yoga and meditation practice, one might be forgiven for concluding that Yoga is primarily concerned with the body, and meditation with the mind. Even to many of its most devoted and accomplished adherents, doing Yoga primarily means pouring the energies of body and breath into a series of postures that can range from soft to strenuous. Few are aware, though, that this dynamic approach was developed mostly in the last millennium or so, and is the still-evolving "baby" in the Yoga family. Its tenth-century creators called it Hatha Yoga—meaning "forceful" or "energy" Yoga—to distinguish it from the "royal" or "highest" path, Rāja Yoga—the cultivation of mental unification, or samādhi, leading to wisdom and liberation. That path had been laid out by Patañjali nearly a thousand years earlier in the definitive text of classical Yoga, the *Yoga Sūtra*. The oldest surviving Hatha Yoga text, dating from the fifteenth century, insists that Hatha and Rāja Yoga were related and were meant to be practiced side by side. Although this decisive instruction is not universally acknowledged, nor followed very closely in most Yoga rooms today, when it is obeyed the relationship of Hatha to Rāja

Yoga becomes clearer, and they may be seen to form a single path with many portals.

This becomes evident not only at the deep end of the Yoga pool but also in the shallows where most of us first dip a toe or two. Yoga does promise—and can quickly deliver—a smorgasbord of physical self-enhancements, to flexibility, strength, health, and beauty, as well as the possibility of dwelling in a relaxed bodily environment with fewer pressures, restrictions, or even clothes, imposed upon bodily form. However, it is the peaceful glow one is likely to feel after even the very first Yoga experience that may bring one back. That ineffable sense of contentment, clarity, and presence can awaken us to the possibility of something far greater, like a trickle of oil bubbling up out of the ground from a vast subterranean reservoir of energy. What may have sprung from the desire to enhance oneself can be transmuted over time into a quest for what lies beyond the self and its desires. It is then that yogis begin to tap the ancient, meditative roots—more likely to be emphasized in Buddhist practice than Yoga at present, at least in the West—and seek to draw upon their enormous stores of knowledge.

At first glance, though, meditation hardly seems to involve the body very much at all. One generally sits still, hushing the lush music of bodily gesture, and contemplates something. While that "something"—the breath or a mantra or perhaps a principle—may be related to or even located in the body, awakening would appear to be about arriving at a fresh, nonordinary, and enlightened understanding. It is difficult for the mind to imagine, much less accept, that this understanding might occur to something other than itself.

As we move beyond these superficial impressions, however, and peer in more closely at both the traditions of yogic liberation and our felt sense of how Yoga actually unfolds in oneself, it may become clearer how misleading and confining these views are. In the process of breaking down false barriers of distinction, the terrain of Yoga cannot help but broaden and perhaps deepen as well. We may even be able to penetrate to the great source, the luminous energy that underlies all practice and lights the way to freedom.

The Tree of Yoga

ROOTS, TRUNK, BRANCHES

It would be an extraordinary thing to be able to follow the traditions of Yoga and meditation back along their branches to the trunk, and perhaps even down to the roots hidden beneath layers of time. But is there any way of knowing where and when Yoga actually began? Despite the hopeful inclination of some today to see yogic practices in the most ancient remnants of the Indus Valley civilization—for example, in four-thousand-year-old clay seals that are often claimed to depict a yogic posture or even a proto-Śiva figure—there is no compelling evidence that any sort of inward-focused, as opposed to god-centered, spiritual tradition existed among either indigenous or migrant peoples of the Indian subcontinent before the beginning of the first millennium B.C.E. Certainly the spirituality of the Aryan tribes that appear to have infiltrated from the northwest and to have come to dominate the area and its cultures throughout the second millennium B.C.E. was heavily materialistic and oriented toward hearing, obeying, and propitiating the gods of a pantheon to rival the Greeks.

There is considerable evidence that by the end of that millennium, a newly expanding capacity of human consciousness for self-awareness and internal motivation had begun to spread in the region. As in other parts of the world, this development gradually superseded the earlier, divinely directed status quo, and likely was related to the widespread social upheaval and fragmentation that characterize this period. In fact, by the seventh or eighth centuries B.C.E. there had developed a broad tolerance and support, sometimes verging on veneration, for a vast counterculture of wandering ascetic spiritual "strivers," or śramaṇa. Rejecting Brahmānical authority, with its relentless sacrifices and rigid hierarchies of race, class, and gender, untold numbers of men and women dropped out, shunning conventional social roles and mores by going forth into homelessness and independent spiritual seeking. Their "inner sacrifices," ranging from harsh austerity to blissful meditation, also began to inform post-Vedic Brahmānical teachings such as the *Upaniṣads*.

The thread that united most of these starkly diverse early Yogas was their intense focus on self-liberation from suffering. Whether through meditative trance, philosophical inquiry, naturalistic observation, hypermorality, or self-mortification, almost all the various approaches operated from a belief that it must be possible somehow for individuals to shake the bonds of misperception that shackled them to an unending cycle of birth and death, saṃsāra—a distinctly non-Aryan worldview. Indeed, since one's salvation lay not in a relationship to external gods but rather in overcoming ignorance (avidyā), one had to transform oneself and one's own perceptions. Even as ascetics clustered around charismatic and compelling seekers such as the Buddha and the Jain Mahāvīra—both emerging from the warrior caste instead of the Brahmān—the prevailing ethos was self-empowering. Regardless of background, liberation was within one's grasp.

Ironically, the spreading tent of the much later Hinduism eventually came, after many centuries, to enclose the unorthodox praxis of Yoga, linking Patañjali to Viṣṇu and installing his teaching as one of the six orthodox philosophical perspectives, or darśana. This has never been a perfect fit, though, Yoga being primarily a path rather than a philosophy, and the *Yoga Sūtra* more a road map than an ontological treatise. It is often forgotten that Patañjala-Yoga shares not only the same basic meditative approach as the Buddha, but also a similar spirit of independence or even anti-orthodoxy. As with the Buddha, Patañjali gently points to the fundamental limitations of a spiritual authority based on revealed texts such as the *Vedas*—and even the *Yoga Sūtra* itself, for that matter—or restricted to any one class or gender. Though later Hindu traditions, eventually including even the countercultural extremes of Hatha Yoga, came to regard it as the essential expression of yogic truth and still look to its 196 lines for inspiration and direction, the radical nature of the *Yoga Sūtra*'s meditative roots has largely been obscured by the intervening centuries and their layers of assimilation, intellectualization, and conflation.

But what of this Patañjali, whose *Yoga Sūtra* is the definitive non-

Buddhist guide to liberation? Although tradition claims he was an important grammarian of the second century B.C.E., more recent scholarly investigations have identified several illustrious Patañjalis and reliably place the author of the *Yoga Sūtra* much later. The work was probably composed between 100 and 300 C.E., but it is now clear that most of its teachings are ancient, based on oral traditions that harken back to a time at least a millennium earlier, and concern the contemplative practices prevalent well before and also after the Buddha (newly corrected dates suggest the Buddha lived roughly from 460 to 380 B.C.E., teaching the Dharma from around 425 B.C.E. on). It is also apparent that by the early centuries of the Common Era the meditative Yoga tradition Patañjali sought to encapsulate in the *Yoga Sūtra* had absorbed many key Buddhist teachings, especially as articulated by later schools such as the Sarvāstivāda (Skt: lit., the teaching that everything is in this moment). It had also begun to question certain elements found in others, for example, what it took to be idealism in the Yogācāra perspective.

Now that the time frame of the Buddha and Patañjali is clearer, and perhaps as well some sense of the interrelated nature of their teachings, one might say that the techniques of Buddhist and yogic meditation form a single braid. The oldest strands—those that predate the Buddha and include practices such as blissful absorptive concentration prevalent among śramaṇa like the Jains—are woven into both the fifth-century B.C.E. Buddha's teachings and also the second-century C.E. *Yoga Sūtra,* where they are in some cases augmented, modified, or refined by later yogic or Buddhist understandings.

The Meditative Yoga of the *Yoga Sūtra*

The shared perspective of these two traditions clearly emerges in the very first lines of the *Yoga Sūtra,* where Patañjali begins by defining Yoga and the universal misperception it resolves:

> Yoga is to still the patterning of consciousness (citta-vṛtti).
> Then pure awareness can abide in its very nature.
> Otherwise awareness takes itself to be the patterns of consciousness.[1]

Stilling reveals something that is generally not seen (avidyā) by human beings, condemning us to suffer: that which actually knows nature in all its manifestations is a timeless, subjectless, unconditioned awareness. Although the mind can imagine and express this awareness as having both a divine universal perspective (Īśvara) and also an individual one (puruṣa), knowing is not an entity or point of view at all, lying beyond the reach of the mind and its insistence on location, orientation, temporality, and attributes. This has riled scholars and religionists who have equated puruṣa with the Ātman—Soul, Self, Seer, Spirit—common to other systems, or confused Patañjali's Īśvara with the divine cause of the universe described in some Hindu texts. This is not surprising, as Patañjali appears to have borrowed the term *puruṣa* and several other concepts from another, even more ancient system, Sāṃkhya, the analytical perspective traditionally if not always accurately paired with the more experiential Yoga, and also bound to be absorbed eventually into Hindu orthodoxy. Sāṃkhya is fundamentally atheistic, and although the *Yoga Sūtra* departs from that to some extent in its description of Īśvara, Patañjali makes clear that puruṣa and Īśvara are beyond causality, attributes, or worship, being nothing more than the unchanging property of knowing immanent in the cosmos. This realization, stripped of all personal, material, or devotional associations, is what will be seen directly—vidyā—as opposed to imagined in the mind when awakening occurs.

In other words, what is important for a suffering being to realize is that it is this imperturbable witnessing that knows, and not one's perceptions, feelings, or thoughts. Every bit of conscious experience, including sensations, emotions, and ideas, issues from contingent body-mind phenomena that are in constant flux and are not "self" in and of themselves. When the pure, unchanging awareness of puruṣa is mistaken for these shifting contents of body or mind, we are not s things as they are (avidyā). Though the inconstancy of their ups downs feels unsettling and personal, in fact, sensations, thoughts, and feelings are nothing more than momentary displays projected as consciousness unfolding before awareness.

This is the great discovery of the ancient Indian yogis: though our bodies and their surroundings may be real, all we can actually know of them are representations appearing as one's consciousness, citta. Each distinct display, also called citta, is a fleeting shadow play involving one of the six types of phenomena: sights, sounds, smells, tastes, tactile feelings, and thought forms. Even though separate and sequential, these cittas unfold so rapidly that we usually misperceive them as an unbroken, simultaneous flow we call "reality," "the world," "me," and "you." This makes it almost impossible to distinguish between mind and matter, or between events and our reactions to them. So our patterns of perception and volition are largely determined, automatic, and nearly inescapable.

How to Do, How to Be

Under ordinary circumstances this illusion of a me navigating myself through a seamless life is virtually impenetrable. But when attention is focused on the processes of body and breath, which orient the yogi in what Patañjali calls Yoga or "yoking," consciousness begins to settle spontaneously and become transparent and reflective, like the ocean growing calm. The meditative intentions that move the yogi down this natural path to tranquillity are twofold. First, the yogi trains himself or herself to keep returning to the point of focus and to sit with it. This intention, called abhyāsa (sit facing), is the basis for sustained practice and begins with witnessing the current stream of bodily sensations. As the yogi keeps noticing and returning from distraction, he quickly comes face-to-face with conditioned habits of thought and reaction. No matter how numerous or overwhelming the distractions, though, they always dissolve unless actively recharged. As they dissipate, the yogi may soon begin to sense a developing aptitude for remembering the focus, a power that starts to grow stronger than his penchant for forgetting it. As this aptitude is cultivated and concentration—samādhi—begins to coalesce, Patañjali points out, the yogi will require only occasional, subtle prompts to direct and train awareness on the object, and the need even for these will drop away as samādhi ripens.

The other intention one must keep in mind if meditation is to move from doing to being is to soften in the midst of what's being experienced. Again and again, the yogi unclenches, relaxes his psychosomatic grip on the moment and allows the events in his chosen field of observation to be just as they are. His success is proportionate to his willingness to let each new impulse to control or improve upon experience simply appear, bloom, and fade. As he does so, it becomes ever clearer that each of his bodily contractions was conditioned by a mental one, arising from desire, aversion, or simply the holding of a self-image in mind. The yogi realizes how much of his mental life has been engaged in reconnoitering on behalf of the self-image for stimulation and gratification. He may also recognize how attaining them never produces anything like a lasting happiness, for the self-image is itself inconstant and can never satisfy, any more than the water in a mirage. This perceptual reeducation, called vairāgya (nonreacting), involves entrusting oneself to one new quantum of experience after another. As each fresh agitation or stab of resistance is recognized and permitted to settle, one unexpectedly notices that familiar sources of disturbance—"triggers"—are no longer having any effect. In this way the yogi realizes that a profound equanimity has quietly developed.

Yoga's Eightfold Path, Aṣṭāṅga

Like most yogis of his time and place, Patañjali appears to have been deeply inspired by the Buddha's teachings, and the *Yoga Sūtra* clearly owes much of its organization and thrust to the Buddhist traditions both ancient and contemporary up to the second or third century. Despite certain differences of philosophical description and emphasis, their yogic paths are virtually indistinguishable, as we shall see, and verbatim quotes abound. Patañjali's path diverges from earlier, non-Buddhist models by adopting the well-known structure of the Buddha's eightfold path (Pali: aṭṭanga-magga), reconfiguring it to be more explicitly about developing dhyāna—or in Pali, jhāna.

YAMA

The first of Yoga's eight aspects or "limbs" is yama. In five pithy lines Patañjali lists "disciplines" that address the yogi's relationship to the world. These depart from the customary precepts—likely familiar to the yogi already—in order not only to inspire but to offer benchmarks for progress:

> Being firmly grounded in nonviolence creates an atmosphere in which others can let go of their hostility.
> For those grounded in truthfulness, every action and its consequences are imbued with truth.
> For those who have no inclination to steal, the truly precious is at hand.
> The chaste acquire vitality.
> Freedom from wanting unlocks the real purpose of existence.[2]

NIYĀMA

The second limb of Yoga is niyāma. These five types of "discipline" are more "internal," yoking different aspects of the yogi's personal sphere to the process of realization:

> With bodily purification, one's body ceases to be compelling, likewise contact with others.
> Purification also brings about clarity, happiness, concentration, mastery of the senses, and capacity for self-awareness.
> Contentment brings unsurpassed joy.

As intense discipline burns up impurities, the body and its senses become supremely refined.
Self-study deepens communion with one's personal deity.
Through orientation toward the divine ideal of pure awareness, Īśvara, one can achieve samādhi.[3]

ĀSANA

As with the Buddha, Patañjali's meditation begins with the body. No elaborate movements are recommended in the third yogic limb, merely a simple sitting posture in which one can relax all physical effort. In fact, āsana derives from the root *ās,* which means "to be here" and also can connote "sitting here." With sustained practice, the first benchmark (samāpatti) of concentration occurs, as the stream of body sensations is recognized as indivisible from the rest of nature—whether internal or external, all experience is projected through the yogi's consciousness. As even beginning meditators can attest, the harsh polarities of self/other and pleasure/pain begin to soften:

The meditation posture (āsana) should embody steadiness and ease (sthira-sukha).
This occurs as all effort relaxes and the first attainment (samāpatti) of samādhi arises, revealing that the body and the infinite universe are indivisible.
Then, one is no longer disturbed by the play of opposites.[4]

As this first meditative practice makes clear, Yoga's eight elements should not be thought of as progressive, like rungs on a ladder, but more like limbs that must interact to carry one forward on the path. Each can mature to the point of transformation, as here samādhi, the eighth limb, blooms directly from āsana, the third.

Of course, many modern treatments of the *Yoga Sūtra* have been written by Hatha Yoga masters understandably inclined to interpret

Patañjali's words "stable" and "easy, comfortable" in line II.46—sthira-sukha—as referring to the "firmness" and "softness" of much later dynamic Hatha Yoga postures such as the Triangle pose. Just a few minutes into sitting meditation, though, it becomes clear that the relaxation of effort Patañjali is advocating here leads to the discovery of increasingly subtle degrees of contraction, which then can be released as well. As if by themselves, extraordinary qualities of steadiness, composure, and bodily pleasure begin to arise. It is significant that, in describing the experience of deepening relaxation and stillness in sitting meditation, the Buddha appears to have used the very same words.

PRĀṆĀYĀMA

With mental images of the body-as-entity starting to dissolve, the yogi can observe a similar progression unfold with energy, or prāṇa, observed manifesting as "breath" in the fourth limb. Becoming attuned to the flow, phase by phase, reveals ever subtler patterns of reaction and resistance that would otherwise trigger more unconscious, automatic patterns. As these become visible, they can be let go, allowing the breath to naturally become softer and less hurried, its duration extended—the literal meaning of āyāma. So, prāṇāyāma in this pre-Hatha teaching is an unforced, natural "breath elongation" that develops the more the yogi lets go. Just "yoking" to this process and letting it ripen is enough to cause the "breathness" of prāṇa to drop away, leaving a luminous or vibratory distillation of consciousness—called nimitta or "characteristic sign" or "counterpart (of consciousness)" in Buddhist teaching—as the pervasive, unifying object or field. When absorption, or dhyāna, fully ripens to its fourth stage, there no longer remains any sense of breathing at all—another phenomenon attested in the Buddhadharma:

> With bodily effort relaxing, the flow of inhalation and exhalation can arrive at a standstill; this is called "breath energy elongation" (prāṇāyāma).

> As the movement patterns of each inhalation, exhalation, and lull are observed—duration, number, and area of focus—breath becomes spacious and subtle.
> In the fourth dhyāna, the distinction between breathing in and out falls away.
> Then the veil lifts from the mind's luminosity.
> And the mind's potential for concentration can be tapped.[5]

Here, too, many interpreters today insist that these lines concern dynamic forms of breath control probably pioneered many centuries later by Tantric Hatha yogis. In fact, with these powerful, relatively newer techniques the yogi can sometimes plunge directly into presence, which is unusually sensitive to the breath energies. It is important to realize that this can happen readily even without the later techniques, though, and both Patañjali and the Buddha clearly indicate that no active effort to control breath, body, or mind remains in the higher stages of dhyāna, which is defined below.

PRATYĀHĀRA, THE WITHDRAWAL OF THE SENSES

Observing one's consciousness of body and breath energies become distilled into a vibrant nimitta epiphenomenon of some kind completely unifies attention, temporarily neutralizing the power of externals to distract:

> When consciousness interiorizes by uncoupling from external objects, the senses do likewise; this is called withdrawal of the senses (pratyāhāra).
> Then the senses reside utterly in the service of realization.[6]

Although this factor is listed fifth, pratyāhāra signals the ripening of all six meditative limbs, as might already have been gleaned from the effects of āsana and prāṇāyāma described above. Patañjali says elsewhere that beyond this turning point, the yogi's perspective becomes more fully interiorized, not unlike the Buddha's powerfully elegant instruction to abide in the "body within the body," explored below.

DHĀRAṆĀ, DHYĀNA, AND SAMĀDHI

Whatever type of object or field the yogi has welcomed or moved to center stage, the progression is the same: the more collected and purified mind becomes, the less hospitable its environment grows for the usually unconscious patterns of physical and mental contraction. The final three limbs of Yoga are a continuum where all names, concepts, psychosomatic structures, and volitions come to subside, after which only a phenomenon's bare arising and passing away remain:

> One-pointedness (dhāraṇā) locks consciousness on a single area.
>
> In meditative absorption (dhyāna), the entire perceptual flow is aligned with that object.
>
> When only the bare qualities of the object shine forth, as if formless, samādhi has arisen.[7]

Discrimination and Freedom

As the eight factors of Yoga mature in samādhi, it starts to become clear that consciousness (citta) does not really know, but is merely a display being known in the emptiness of pure awareness (puruṣa). The discriminating insight (viveka) that recognizes the difference is not an idea but something that must be directly seen. This direct vision (vidyā), possible when the relentless agitations of mental and physical reactivity have calmed to crystal clarity, is what sees through the everyday misidentification (avidyā) that produces the illusory sense of "I," whose wanting, not wanting, and self-preservation underlie all human suffering:

> As soon as one can distinguish between consciousness (citta) and awareness (puruṣa), the ongoing construction of the self ceases.
>
> Consciousness, now oriented to this distinction (viveka), can gravitate toward freedom—the fully integrated knowledge that awareness is empty and of a different order than unfolding nature.[8]

This now utterly nondiscursive Yoga terminates in the direct vision (vidyā) and knowledge (prajñā) that suffering is nothing more than an artifact of consciousness. Unconditioned knowing, whether conceived subsequently on a universal and divine scale (Īśvara) or on an individual one (puruṣa), is untouched by change, uncolored by suffering, impersonal, timeless.

One who regards even the most exalted states disinterestedly, discriminating continuously between pure awareness and the phenomenal world, enters the final stage of integration, in which nature is seen to be a shower of irreducible experiential states (dharma-megha). This realization extinguishes both the causes of suffering and the cycle of cause and effect.

Once all the layers and imperfections concealing truth have been washed away, insight is boundless, with little left to know. Then the seamless flow of reality, its transformations colored by the fundamental qualities of nature (guṇā), begins to break down, fulfilling the true mission of consciousness.

> One can see that the flow is actually a series of discrete events, each corresponding to the merest instant of time, in which one form becomes another. Freedom (kaivalya) is at hand when the fundamental qualities of nature, each of their transformations witnessed at the moment of its inception, are recognized as irrelevant to pure awareness; it stands alone, grounded in its very nature, the power of pure seeing.[9]

Though awareness has been designated "puruṣa" and lingui cast as an entity, it is not even an "it," being naturally of a different order, standing apart (kaivalya) from the constructs of birth, identity, thought, and experience, with which the yogi had previously confused it. Although most of his inherited and acquired personal attributes will continue to some extent, they are joined by the postcessation fruitional knowledge (prajñā) that they're mere processes. Even though spinning like juggler's plates, held up by the momentum of some earlier push, they're doomed to topple before long.

Thus, the yogi has not become free from anything—awareness was already free, awaiting recognition from a purified consciousness. Not unlike the power in Dorothy's ruby slippers, the path to awakening is waiting within us, ready to appear when mind is brought together with some aspect of unfolding reality and yoked to it persistently enough for the dizzying dramas of self to dissipate. The yogi now feels an unprecedented security in the impersonal and impermanent: there's no place like home.

The Yoga of the Buddha

A careful exploration of the Buddha's Yoga, both through practice and analysis, finds it virtually indistinguishable from the praxis elucidated by the *Yoga Sūtra*. Like Patañjali, the Buddha was highly pragmatic, as we shall see, but his central style of practice is no less a Yoga of energy than the āsana-prāṇāyāma approach described above. One need look no farther than Buddha's name for it, *ānāpānasati,* a Pali compound rendered as *prāṇa-apāna-smṛti* in Sanskrit Buddhist texts. Ānāpānasati means "remembering [to be aware as] energy flows down and up." Many Yoga practitioners will be familiar with the terms *prāṇa* and *apāna,* identified with the influx and outflow of what we today call breath. It's important for modern practitioners to look beyond the modern conceptualization of this as respiration, however, in which the yogi practices "mindfulness of breathing." To the early yogis, respiration was not conceived as a physiological process so much as one of the ways that the life force or vital energy—prāṇa—pervading all creation could be perceived directly. Breathing is therefore the experience of prāṇa as a specific tidal pattern infusing the whole being, and not limited to the respiratory apparatus. The early yogis discovered that training themselves to experience this energy's movements with growing awareness and precision—what the Buddha called a "body in the body"—brought about a more intimate and wise connection—presence, or upaṭṭhāna in Pali, upasthāna in Sanskrit—with unfolding reality. Since its movements are ever changing and can only be felt in the present moment, prāṇa and apāna comprise a powerful and reliable avenue to knowing things as they are, right now.

Furthermore, this path leading from the body to its experience as energy is available to the yogi at all times, as long as life and breath continue. However, in the beginning yogis can hardly be conscious enough, despite their best efforts, to avoid forgetting where they are and repeatedly falling back on the usual, everyday bodily and mental patterns that comprise our illusory but very convincing sense of self. Because the body is energetic by nature, each time the yogi "remembers" (sati) the possibility of presence in the bodily form, the tides of prāṇa or apāna are there for the observing, just as the source of a spring continually produces a fresh stream of waves and ripples. The Yoga of directing and maintaining one's attention on this source, whatever the "field"—the Buddha used the remarkable phrase yoniso manasikāra, or "keeping attention right where things are being born"—orients the yogi to the present moment. Furthermore, it sensitizes him to recognize and let go of each mental structure—such as memory, imagination, or self-feeling—that attempts to pass for reality.

As might be growing evident, the heart of this "Yoga of liberation," as we might call both Patañjali's path and the Buddha's, is seeing (Pali: vijjā; Skt: vidyā, related to both the Latin and the modern word *video*). Both Patañjali and the Buddha carefully and repeatedly instructed their followers to regard seeing as the primary means by which human beings can come to freedom. The root cause of suffering, the primary kleśa or affliction in the *Yoga Sūtra* is avidyā (Pali: avijjā), or "not seeing." Specifically, human beings generally fail to recognize that awareness itself is empty of characteristics or reactions, not unlike space, and therefore already free. Though the Buddha famously identified craving (tanhā) as the cause of suffering—the principle he called the Second Noble Truth—he also traced craving and its consequences back to their source in avijjā/avidyā in his later analysis of the conditioned, impersonal processes that support the illusion of selfhood, namely dependent origination (paticca-samuppāda).

Although commonly translated as "ignorance," avijjā/avidyā does not actually mean that one lacks some special information that, once acquired by the mind, will produce awakening and freedom of the heart. Broad or deep though one's knowledge may be—of wisdom teachings, scientific findings, or logic—there is no guarantee of, or even correlation to, what the Buddha called seeing things as they are. It is important to stay within the true meaning of vijjā/vidyā as "direct seeing," which only applies to what is actually in front of one right now, at this very moment. Both Yoga and dharma arise in the profound recognition that this moment is the only reality, and therefore all one can truly know and work with.

As we saw earlier, the actual meaning of vidyā is underscored by Patañjali in the *Yoga Sūtra* when he identifies the two poles of the yogic will as abhyāsa and vairāgya. Abhyāsa literally means "being with what's in front of you right now." Abhyāsa is worth breaking down. *Abhi* means "toward," and it also carries the sense of "higher" or "superior." *As* is a verb root meaning "to be here," in the sense of existing in the present moment; its secondary meaning, usually positioned in dictionaries as the primary, more usual one, is "to sit." This makes sense—in everyday life, when something is right here, it's usually sitting here, so the root *as* is the platform for words like "sitting posture" and even "chair" or "throne." To Patañjali, however, abhyāsa means the practice of repeatedly turning toward and facing what is before one right now.

After all one cannot see something that one isn't facing, and the moment it's not here, the only way to "see" it is to remember it or to imagine it, once again turning away from what is here right now. Each time we forget that the "events" unfolding in memory and imagination are not really happening now, we are once again caught up in identification and no longer seeing things as they are.

THE INTENTION TO AWAKEN

Likewise for the Buddha, the practice is centered around seeing in the present moment. When the yogi turns attention to the body, he or she is unlikely to see it as it really is in its elemental form (yathā bhūta), namely, a complex stream of impersonal matter animated by various mental and physical actions that are largely conditioned and subliminal. Instead, the yogi will initially experience the body as solid, personal, and enduring—namely, "me." What the yogi must do, though, is begin to study it more closely.

The yogi abides observing the body within the body (kāye kāya), remembering (satimā) to be intensely (ātāpi) present and immediately aware (sampajāno).

The most essential yogic act to enable a deeper knowing is to remember—one must remember to keep at it so that the quality of seeing can develop and clarify. The Buddha's key word, *sati,* is usually translated as "mindfulness," but literally means "memory," and in this context is a skillful means that in the late stages of awakening will no longer be required.

Once the yogi resolves to sit in meditation and awaken, the first instance of sati is remembering to form an intention, expressed by a phrase attributed to the Buddha, parimukhaṃ satiṃ upaṭṭhapetvā.[10] Although some traditions have understood this phrase to mean that the yogi "establishes mindfulness around the face," *parimukhaṃ* usually means what's "ahead" or "in front." In other words, the Buddha is asking the yogi to remember what lies ahead and to form a clear intention. We know that this intention is of vital importance because the Buddha advises the yogi that awakening requires the quality of ātāpa—an of will to both see and surrender that requires a strong initial sustained by disciplined "remembering." Furthermore, experien that attempts to arrive at clear seeing tend to founder without it.

THE CURRENT OF PRĀṆA

Once this intention is established, the yogi is to become aware that prāṇa and apāna are indeed flowing at this very moment. This current is to be the basis for each of the Buddha's four key instructions leading to the refined seeing (vidyā) of what is happening now that leads to the end of suffering. The first aspect—that which most readily becomes tangible—is the direction of the flow.

> The yogi is mindful as breath flows in, mindful as breath flows out.[11]

The yogi begins by remembering—sati—to refresh awareness each time the flowing energy of breath changes directions. It is important to understand that the Buddha is not saying "be aware of the breath." Instead, he's saying "be aware—directly and immediately—of the energy of this current only." That fact, generally overlooked, is of the greatest importance because it cuts like a razor to the very heart of the misperception that grants one's "I," or self-feeling, its illusory sense of continuity. For most beginning yogis, ordinary breathing has long since dropped from the screen of conscious awareness and therefore only exists subliminally except in times of respiratory distress. As such, its behaviors and their relation to other bodily and mental behaviors are almost completely hidden from normal view.

When the yogi attempts to observe the breath, he may first encounter a sense of the "whole breath"—breathing in and out—as a repetitive and relatively uniform rhythmic event. As he studies each distinct flow, however, a more nuanced sense emerges. The duration of a "whole breath" is simply too long for it to be experienced except as a composite, a mental mirage unconsciously produced by short-term memory. Absent that mode of remembering, one can only be aware of the momentary feelings of the current—mere instants in the arc of a single flow. At any time from that point on, the yogi may suddenly notice that the "I" of self-feeling is no different.

As soon as the vague outline of "now flowing in" and "now flowing out" become observable to the yogi, the Buddha's second instruction can then begin: to know that the current is long as it unfolds long, and short when short.

> As breath flows in or out for a long time, the yogi is aware how long; as breath flows in or out for a short time the yogi is aware how short.[12]

The Buddha is suggesting that one can know directly—pajānāti, a verb form of paññā/prajñā—as opposed to merely thinking how long each breath takes to transpire. Under ordinary circumstances, the most likely, if not necessarily self-evident, way to gauge the length of the breath is to unconsciously control it and then mentally label the span as "long" or "short." This is not the intention, however, nor does the yogi need to quantify the duration of each breathflow by, for example, timing it with a stopwatch. What is being offered here is the possibility of greater intimacy and presence in the momentarily flowing energy that comprises the "body in the body" (kāye kāya). In the famous simile, which may or may not have originated with the Buddha himself, this process is compared to a craftsman turning a lathe or pottery wheel. As the object—clay, for example—rapidly spins, the potter applies a finger or tool at some point and slowly moves along, then lifts it away. Clearly the potter's sense of how long this turn or "pass" lasted derives from the sensations of actual contact from the beginning of the pass, through the middle to the end. It's being present and aware of the continuity of contact, and not some mental conception of the "whole," by which the potter knows the long and short of it directly (pajānāti).

Nor does the yogi need to establish or become entrained in a rhythm

—in fact, the opposite. The experience of a rhythm requires a mental action "putting together" (saṅkhāra/saṃskāra) at least two durations, and the instructions explicitly are about confining one's attention simply to the flow happening now. In the Buddhist approach, the yogi is to let go of deliberate breathing, and therefore has no way of knowing how long the next current will be. He must therefore observe the actual sensations that are making contact with awareness moment by moment from beginning to middle to end.

With these two simple but profound instructions—observe only the current direction of flow and sense its duration through sustained contact—the Buddha has led even the least sophisticated yogi to a profound, face-to-face encounter with the bodily energies of this moment, narrowing the window of observation to the unfolding present. The usual, everyday mode of observation unconsciously entails thinking, analysis memory, anticipation, emotional reactions, and other mental and physical responses. But by simply focusing on the unfolding body energies of the current flow, and knowing them as they unfold from the beginning of one flow until the end, the Buddha has laid the foundation for the two most important instructions—how the yogi is to now "train" himself—sikkhati—to see things as they are:

> The yogi trains himself to experience the whole body as breath flows in, then to experience the whole body as breath flows out.
>
> The yogi trains oneself to relax bodily activity as breath flows in, then to relax bodily activity as breath flows out.[13]

In the first of the two trainings, the Buddha now instructs the yogi to remember the possibility—sati—of experiencing the "whole body"—sabba-kāya—directly just during the duration of the prevailing current, to which he or she has become sensitized. But what did the Buddha mean exactly by the "whole body"? Although the answer to this question may seem self-evident, it has aroused much controversy in the various Buddhist traditions. The relevant Pali commentaries conclude, rather oddly, that by "body" he actually meant the breath phase itself, with "whole" referring to its duration. However, the yogi has already been doing this very thing. These commentaries and some later teachers insist that the Buddha must have meant this, though, since in the *Ānāpānasati Sutta* he refers to the breathflow as "a body among the bodies,"[14] which they claim supports the idea that the breath is the "body in the body" that is the basis of satipaṭṭhāna as well as the referent for the "whole body."

Relying on pronouncements found in one or two other sūttas to argue these kinds of points turns out to be a risky business, however. Today we have no reliable idea what the true contexts were for many of the key discourses—it is doubtful, for example, that the Buddha ever traveled as far as Delhi, the purported setting for the *Satipaṭṭhāna Sutta,* a key discourse in which these instructions appear—much less which of the words attributed to the Buddha are actually his, since none of them are in the Ardha-Magadhi dialect he himself appears to have spoken. Although the various recensions of the Canon that we have today in full or in part—Theravāda, Sarvāstivāda, Dharmaguptaka, MulaSarvāstivāda, Mahāsaṅghika—present a philosophical edifice that appears astonishingly coherent and consistent considering its scope, a close examination reveals not only countless discrepancies but also abundant evidence that the Buddha's circle and their immediate followers in the presectarian period following his death were often unclear about what he had meant. Their attempts to arrive at ironclad definitions and thereby "close the book" on key phrases such as "the whole body" and "bodily formations" appear to be unmistakable signs of disagreement. It seems that the Buddha, acting out of pragmatism and wisdom, was often careful to avoid specifics, both when describing the nature of things as he saw it and even more so when prescribing a course of action. This, more than any other single factor, may account for much of the doctrinal squabbling, sectarianism, and one-upsmanship prevalent in succeeding generations, and even to some extent the eventual rise of Mahāyāna, Vajrayāna, and Zen.

BHĀVANĀ

TO DEVELOP AND "MAKE MUCH OF"

To understand why the Buddha may have meant exactly what he said about "experiencing the whole body." it may be helpful to consider how the path of observing the body starts in one place and, like all paths worth following, leads to another. This is the case when Patañjali, deeply familiar with the Buddha's approach, broke down this approach into how asana develops from relaxing the whole body to knowing it as energy currents.

An aspect of meditation that the Buddha never tired of pointing out, in fact, is its progressive nature. This is typified by his use of the word *bhāvanā* (development) to describe the trajectory of realization. Each practice sits along a continuum of bhāvanā, connecting the initial conditioned "everyday" state or dhamma to those in which the practice has been fully realized and "made much of." Thus, the Buddha is not waxing philosophical—his only concern is whether the practice works. Yogis, meanwhile, are to adjust their approach as necessary in order to keep progressing along this continuum toward clarity. For example, as we saw above, the yogi starts meditating by observing the body in its conventional sense, replete with unseen but karmically active mental structures of past, future, "I," and "mine." Except in extraordinary circumstances, where extreme pain, danger, or other intense conditions plunge one into presence, yogis have little choice but to begin practice with the ordinary, everyday delusions—that they are their thoughts, that the remembered or owned body of identity is the actual body in form. In other words, at first the body is just a body—a solid entity that is "mine." But kāya is really more like the word *body* in its group connotation—a "legislative body," say, or a "body of evidence." Yogis' discernment of the body moves along this continuum, starting with the body's initial appearance as a single entity and clarifying until they sense the "body in the body"—the unfolding, ever-changing energies (āna/prāṇa and apāna) that are arising and passing away in each current, and then even more quickly, with each fleeting moment of contact as awareness expands to include all sensory-mental phenomena.

The perception of instantaneous arising and passing away, in turn, is the threshold crossing over into Vipassanā, the direct "seeing through" that teases apart the unsatisfactoriness and impermanence—duḥkha-anicca—of all constructive mental and physical events, and the impersonality—anatta—of phenomena. These are the three characteristics of being that are visible with the discernment, or cakṣu-darśana—the "dharma eye"—that is near the terminus (nibbāna/nirvāṇa) in this continuum of clear knowing.

RIGHT EFFORT

Moving along the continuum of development (bhāvanā), many seasoned meditators have arrived at a pair of initially dismaying discoveries: using the same approach every time they sit produces variable results, and the most effective way to become present in any given instance is often a departure from their teacher's instructions. The Buddha seems to have encountered this among his earliest students, and described several different types of temperaments and responses to practice. He is also portrayed in a sizable number of mindfulness teachings as pragmatic and contextual, such as when instructing Sona in the *Satipaṭṭhāna Sutta* to fine-tune his meditation as if he were playing the vīṇā, a sitarlike instrument whose strings may be found either too tight or too loose. When experiencing too much tension while trying to concentrate on a particular object, one can relax the exclusivity and open up to a wider field; likewise, if the quality of presence and immediacy is flagging, one might focus more sharply and energetically. The Buddha seems to be careful to avoid being too specific with Sona, and is similarly vague in the neighboring sutta about the king's favorite cook, whose success stems from arriving at the appropriate balance of ingredients for each new meal.

As the particular properties and processes of each meditation—the "meal" or "tune"—begin to be recognized as unique, evolving as the yogi adjusts the approach, he or she may come to a more flexible and intuitive approach to what the Buddha called "right effort." Right effort is the central axis of meditative development, or bhāvanā, where the yogi practices to bring about what is skillful or conducive to awakening, and to foster it; and also to let go of what is unskillful, and not get caught up in it again. The Buddha distinguishes right effort from the usual things we do when seeking happiness, however; instead, right effort derives from four simple forms of knowing: knowing what leads to vision and surrender; knowing what sustains it; knowing how to let go of what leads away from vision and surrender; and knowing how to prevent it. Unlike the usual efforts to resist, gratify, or escape our burning dissatisfactions, none of these is a typical or automatic response (saṅkhāra/saṃskāra)—they represent a new approach in which the growing capacity to drop our resistance and open up to experience will allow the fires to put themselves out.

Although the Buddha indicated that the process of awakening is developmental and progressive, many traditions have seen fit to "cut to the chase" when observing the "body within the body" as described in instructions above. Teachers both ancient and contemporary have ignored the phrase "whole body" (sabba-kāya) or taken it to mean the breath phase itself, as we saw above, and led yogis to focus on one small area such as the tip of the nose, the upper lip, or the abdomen from the beginning. Indeed, when one begins by feeling the whole bodily field of energies one breathflow at a time, before long the yogi may intuitively lock onto a single, smaller field that is more vivid, pleasant, compelling, or stabilizing, thereby leading to increasingly absorbed states of concentration (jhāna/dhyāna). Thus, it would seem to make sense to fasten on to a more specific field right at the start.

Although this isn't necessarily unskillful, the Buddha himself does not appear to have recommended it. The reason may have to do with the fact that the unfolding practice of observing the body, like all of the states or dhamma that the Buddha describes, is based on bodily conditions that change from moment to moment, hour to hour, day to day. At first, most yogis benefit from feeling a larger field of awareness and observing. And as one peruses the field of the whole body, a particularly important factor that powerfully conduces toward awakening begins to become accessible and therefore workable. This factor is called "investigation" (dhamma-vicaya).

Gathering Energy

To understand dhamma-vicaya, it is helpful to examine the word *vicaya*. The root *ci* means "to gather," and refers to the act of selecting and gathering objects based on their quality, such as firewood or the right stones to build a wall or foundation. When one goes out into the forest to gather wood, very little thinking is required in order to distinguish seasoned pieces, likely to burn well and supply energy, from green; and with experience the process becomes ever simpler. As we have seen, meditative progress depends on making the right kind of effort, which is based on the skill of recognizing the wholesome and letting go of the unwholesome, much like the wood or, say, the cook's ingredients.

To continue the former analogy, if one wished to gain a better sense of where to look for wood, one might move to higher ground in order to survey the whole forest and locate areas with more fallen trees. In the same way, when one "takes in" the whole body, one begins to sense the intuitive way this process of discrimination might zero in on those areas within the greater field of the whole body (sabba-kāya) that are discovered to be more concentration-worthy. Instead of imposing or even choosing an object, the yogi begins to notice that the field or object presents or "selects" itself to some degree.

Within and Without

The yogi may also become aware that under certain conditions the most energetic or engaging phenomena available happen to lie outside the sphere of the body. For example, the evolving qualities of sound or sight may provide a more powerful and stabilizing "surface" on which to see the unfolding present: in other words, external to oneself (bahiddhā) instead of within (ajjhatta).

> In this way the yogi abides observing the body in the body regarding experience within, without, or both.[15]

As vision clarifies and awareness first begins to discern the energetic, impermanent nature of being a body, this same nature can start to be recognized in other sensory and also mental phenomena. The cognitive structures that had compartmentalized existence into "me" and "the world around me" likewise cease to seem ultimate or enduring, and instead merely appear momentary and contingent on mental fabrication (saṅkhāra/saṃskāra). One recalls the way Patañjali described āsana:

> This occurs as all effort relaxes and the first attainment (samāpatti) of samādhi arises, revealing that the body and the infinite universe are indivisible.[16]

It should be noted that most scholastics and monastics seem to have agreed with the improbable notion that by "internal" and "external" the Buddha here meant "in oneself" and "in somebody else." There are a few places in the various recensions where the Buddha does use these words in that sense, but not in the satipaṭṭhāna instructions, where he has just advised the yogi to remove himself from the company of others and practice in solitude. Again and again in the suttas the Buddha describes how the four domains of satipaṭṭhāna, the basic arenas for the development (bhāvanā) of mindfulness (sati), set the stage for profound absorptive states of concentration (jhāna/dhyāna) best cultivated when off by oneself. This is in fact how the Buddha's personal practice is always depicted.

This is not to say that the commentarial understanding—that "external" here means "in someone else"—is without value, however. In the context of a meditative community (saṅgha) or group retreat, mindfulness of others and their energies is one of the most important aspects of practice regarding action, taking its place alongside mindfulness of the bodily positions, movements, and daily activities, since in that context many of these tend to take place in the vicinity of others.

NO "THERE" THERE

The final stages of Buddhist insight, echoed in those described by Patañjali at the end of the *Yoga Sūtra*'s third and fourth chapters, are the awakening of a radical new perspective. More and more, the unfolding reality of "oneself" existing in a "world" is recognized as a parade of inconceivably brief "contacts" (phassā). These tend to trigger karmically active responses (saṅkhāra/saṃskāra) that are inherently neither permanent nor satisfying. Usually, since these qualities of impermanence (anicca) and inability to satisfy (duḥkha) cannot be observed, they stamp experience with the pervasive feeling that it is happening to "oneself," an enduring entity without whom life is unthinkable and who therefore must be preserved at all costs. This puts one at odds with the actual unfolding of life, in which each new moment is unique, and what was is no longer. One doesn't have to be an astrophysicist, envisioning a cosmos that seems to still be expanding outward from an ancient Big Bang, to ponder the fact that every bit of matter is in motion, both externally and in its most subatomic aspects. What had been stardust is now this page, the finger that turns it, and the visual sense watching both.

The yogi abides observing how phenomena—dhamma—arise contingently in the body, or how they pass away, or how they arise and pass away.

As with Patañjali's "shower of irreducible experiential states" in *Yoga Sūtra* IV.29, the Buddhist yogi begins to perceive that the rapidity, brevity, and sheer profusion of these momentary perceptual contacts are increasing. This is not because they actually are, though. Reality has always been like this: a mosaic of discrete phenomena, for which some assembly (saṅkhāra/saṃskāra) has always been required. From any other point of view than the mind's, they are no more than momentary conditions of energy.

PRĀṆA

THE THREAD OF LIBERATIVE YOGA

If Patañjali were to drop in on a Yoga class today, he might not recognize very much of it as Yoga. His stretch of the yogic path moves directly from the pulsating world at large to the subtlest, most fleeting and ineffable aspects of experience knowable. The terminus of this path is consciousness stilled to cessation (nirodha), leaving at least an instant of unconditioned knowing with which one's conditioned processes of self and consciousness will never again be confused. This doesn't happen very often in the Dog pose, or any of the other familiar moves we undertake in Yoga rooms around the world.

So, when we're on the mat, are we really doing Yoga? Yes, even if not in a way that brings us to the brink of liberation. It's no accident that dynamic Hatha Yoga has become the most popular style in the world: it's not only accessible but very powerful. As many in our cerebral modern age have discovered, physical movement is a far more welcoming portal to concentration and mindfulness than "cold" sitting. Even if they generally lie beyond the threshold of stillness necessary for the terminal stages of samādhi, the techniques of "energy Yoga" can quickly expose much of our conditioned mind-body patterning and lay a channel for us to flow toward sitting and samādhi. Working with prāṇa vividly reminds us that dharma practice has always been susceptible to intellectualization, or "dryness," even though there can be no doubt that the Buddha, like Patañjali, taught an experiential Yoga grounded in the energy stream (ānāpāna/prāṇa-apāna) and pointed toward the liberation inherent in knowing all things at their most real.

Whether one is engaged in dynamic Hatha Yoga or the process of cessation (nirodha) realized as the deepest possible sitting stillness, the worlds within and without come to comprise a nondual arena for observing one's own nature. As vision (vidyā) clarifies, the yogi ceases to be misled by the mirages of bodily or mental fabrication (saṅkhāra/saṃskāra), their false distinctions of "body" and "mind," or the appearance of continuity they impart to the confabulated sense of "me."

Instead, the yogi harnesses his or her attention—the primary thrust of Yoga's root concept, yuj—to the aliveness of the field intuitively chosen to work with, be it skin, muscles, joints, fascia, breathflow, the whole body, or the world pouring in through the senses.

The thread uniting these seemingly disparate entities is their nature as prāṇa—energy. In a relative universe, energy may be experienced subjectively as matter, but the yogi's vision is yoked to the movement of unfolding, of arising and passing away, as will be recalled in the Buddha's vivid image, yoniso manasikāra—"keeping attention right where things are being born."[17] This is the only way to know them directly and in their elemental state: not as things at all, but as the contingent, unfolding dharma.

2

BODY AND MIND DROPPED AWAY

ROSHI PAT ENKYO O'HARA

When I first began Zen practice, I read the root manual of Zen meditation by the Japanese master Dōgen. The "Fukanzazengi"[1] starts with enticing phrases about the possibility of "emancipation," and finding our "original self" by stepping back and "turning the light inward." I recall vividly my excitement as I read these opening phrases, anticipating the instructions I so desired in order to discover how to use my mind to change my life. And then, in the next section, as the instructions began, I was surprised, and somewhat deflated, to read the detailed guidance about how to hold the body, to sit, to hold one's hands, feet, mouth, ears, eyes, as well as what kind of cushion to use, clothes to wear, and so on. All of this physical data, and I was looking for the secret of what to do with my mind!

And of course, that was right where I was stuck, thinking that there was a mind practice that did not involve my body, as if my mind were some kind of balloon that floated over me, rather than being integral to every part of my being. Or alternatively, that my body was some kind of chariot that carried my mind around. Either way, I was certainly stuck.

But not uniquely so. At the first retreat center where I practiced, there was little attention paid to posture, as long as one did not move and distract others. Later, when I studied under the Japanese Zen master Maezumi Roshi for over a year I was constantly corrected for my slumping, imbalanced posture—or was it for my slumping, imbalanced thinking? I had not yet learned that they were two ends of the same stick. During much of this correction, I thought, "Oh, that's just my body—what's the problem?"

Just the Body

There is an old story about Dōgen as a young monk visiting China. On a cold and dark morning, he was sitting in deep meditation and was stunned when his teacher, walking behind him, removed a cloth slipper and slapped the dozing monk sitting next to him, saying, "Meditation is not sleeping! Drop away body and mind!"[2] Young Dōgen, at that very moment, experienced a great release. Based on his subsequent teaching, we can guess that he discovered that he was pitched into a state of being where all conceptions of body and mind drop away, and what is left is . . . this moment, in all of its ecstatic, crushing, wondrous liveliness, and its inevitable evaporation.

Some scholars say Dōgen misunderstood that phrase, "drop away body and mind," that actually his teacher, speaking in Chinese, said something like wipe away the dust of the mind. But what Dōgen heard became his core teaching on meditation and on life itself: "Dropping away body and mind, body and mind, dropped away." This phrase in turn became a key way of describing zazen, Zen meditation.[3]

Seven hundred and fifty years later, a middle-aged woman walks on the snow in upstate New York during a long meditation retreat. As my boot sinks through the crust, through layers of ice and snow to the muddy earth below, my foot, my leg, my whole being lets go, drops, body and mind, earth and sky, being and nonbeing. As the old poet Han Shan said,

> There is a body—there is not a body;
> This is me—then again it is not.[4]

This dropping of all concept of body and mind is like a distorting lens falling away and what is left is a realization that I am the snow, the ice, the earth and sky, while I have not stopped being myself.

Once a student asked me if Dōgen's "dropping away body and mind" meant that we should ignore our bodies, not pay any attention to them, numb them? In dropping away body and mind an instruction to ignore the presence of "body awareness" or "mind awareness," to numb out? Or isn't it rather a teaching to drop all conceptions of body and mind? Isn't to drop to release, to let go of our grasping after abstractions? What would happen if there were no positing of "this is body" and "this is mind"—then what would be left? Without the conception "body" there is just this soft whooshing of sensation, internal and external, of muscle, of skin, of feelings, there is flow. Why would we want to block it out? It is our life!

And when there is pain, there too is the flow of our life. A serious dharma student, suffering from knee pain during a retreat, once told me that she had mastered the art of blocking all feeling in her hips, knees, and feet during zazen! What she had found was a way for her mind to obliterate the bottom half of her body. This is not dropping, this is blocking. She threw out the bottom half of her being, the bottom half of her true nature, of her potential to wake up. When there is pain, physical or emotional, there is an opportunity to investigate thoroughly our own being and the source of our pain and the nature of it. Blocking the pain creates a black box of pain, unknown and unchangeable. Moving toward the feeling, we realize that it is fluid, that it has time and motion and variability. We no longer have stuck our pain in a vault, but we meet it with attention and aliveness. How is it possible to engage in a meditation practice of "waking up" by means of blocking the reality of the moment? To deny our reality blinds us from the world itself, from all beings and experiences everywhere.

When we try to control and separate our experience, we miss so much. Earnest seekers often stumble over the truth they are scrambling for. A Zen master walking with his student on a spring day said, "Do you smell the olive blossoms?" "Yes, Teacher." The master replied, "You see, I am hiding nothing from you."[5] Imagine the student's response: "Is this a mystical teaching? What does he mean 'he is hiding nothing?' What is it about the olive blossoms? What do they signify?" He offered his student everything. The fragrance of olive blossoms in spring doesn't lead to some special state, any more than meditation, zazen, or study leads to something other than what is always here, if we can but drop away our preconceptions.

This is beautifully evoked by a story about two early Chinese Zen masters, Nanyue and Mazu. One day Master Nanyue saw Mazu in the courtyard sitting earnestly in meditation. He asked Mazu what he was doing and Mazu said he was sitting zazen in order to attain Buddhahood—awakening. Nanyue then sat down in front of Mazu and began to rub a tile with a rock. Mazu blinked, looked at Nanyue, and asked the obvious, "Why are you rubbing that tile with a rock?" Nanyue kept rubbing and said, "I'm making a mirror." Mazu said, "How can you make a mirror out of tile and rock?" Nanyue replied, "How can you make a Buddha out of sitting in meditation?" Mazu was taken aback, his entire ordering of things fell away, and he whispered, "Master, what then is right?"

That phrase, "What then is right?," is so endearing, in its innocence and direct openness to a new way to realize reality. What then is right? To help Mazu to see for himself, Nanyue resorted to an old saying, "When there is a cart that won't move, do you hit the ox or hit the cart?"[6] As Dōgen has pointed out, the implication of this question itself is marvelous: what do we mean by the cart "not moving"? Is it "not moving" and therefore not part of the flow of impermanence that is an aspect of all creation? Or is it not moving in relation to the ox? Or in relation to some third thing? What would that be?[7]

The richness of this Zen parable lies in its subtle waves of meaning. On one level, Nanyue is showing Mazu that it is not the body that needs to be urged but the mind that must turn. On another level, we could consider what it would be to hit the cart, to urge the body to "move" that is, to manifest the becoming of Buddhahood. Wouldn't it be to take the posture, to take the traditional cross-legged, upright, living form of meditation, and thus to become a Buddha in that act? That's hitting the cart. Or is it the ox? Are they two?

As for Mazu, he was speechless. Nanyue, taking pity on Mazu, explained, "Are you sitting meditation in order to become a Buddha or to sit meditation? If you are sitting to practice meditation, you know that it has nothing to do with sitting or lying down; if you sit to become a Buddha, the Buddha has no fixed form. In this transient, nonabiding world, do not discriminate. If you are practicing to become a Buddha, you kill the Buddha; if you are attached to meditation, you have not yet entered the principle."

It was as if Mazu had breathed the air of life for the first time. It is said that for him it was like drinking delicious ghee. He was able to drop off his ideas and split off notions of discipline, of doing-in-order-to, of grasping for perfection or Buddha. At once Mazu received this powerful instruction: it is not the body, it is not the mind; it is you.

What is this "you"? Returning to the meditation manual I mentioned at the beginning, the Fukanzazengi tells us to learn to step back and turn the light inward, to illuminate the self. Then body and mind drop off naturally, and original self will manifest. What is left when our ideas of body and mind slip away? Right now, what comes to mind is this July moment in the countryside of New York, and so I write,

> The air so damp with heat
> even the mosquito rests,
> silent humming.

One answer to the question of what is left when body and mind drop away is the wholeness of life right here. Right now, while reading this, take a moment to just stop, look up, and breathe in and breathe out, and whatever sounds and smells and worlds are right now swirling around you is what is left when it all drops.

In another chapter of Dōgen's writings, "Zenki," Dōgen likens one's life to riding in a boat; you row, you adjust the rudder and sails, and it is the boat that gives you the ride, and without it, you can't ride. But, he says, "Your riding makes the boat what it is."[8] Again, dropping the separation between body and mind, between boat and sailor, we go directly into the life of the boat. It is the living of your life in your body and mind that makes you who you are. And actualizing one's life through living it brings us back to a realization of our whole being. The Christian mystic Thomas Merton described this experience as no longer being involved in the measurement of one's life "but in the living of it."[9] Merton directs us to a vital aspect of union of body and mind: the living of life as opposed to the theorizing and narrating of it. What makes this living of it possible? Merton found it in prayer, and Dōgen found it in zazen. Here Dōgen expresses this quality of body and mind gathered together:

> In the heart of the night,
> the moonlight framing
> a small boat drifting,
> tossed not by the waves
> nor swayed by the breeze.[10]

There is no struggle here. The boat drifts, and is not pulled this way and that by the waves and the wind. It is the natural flow of meditation, when the struggle is dropped, the mind is not telling the body to perform in any way, nor is the mind struggling against itself to be any way.

This is what is called jijuyu samādhi, the samādhi, or union, of the self receiving and enjoying itself. Imagine the ease of one's whole being giving and receiving to itself, fulfilling itself through its completion. This expression of body and mind meditation renounces all ideas of forcing ourselves to perform a practice and instead offers an image of the ease and natural spontaneity with which a child raises her arm, or a man leans against a tree.

Of course, it doesn't always feel that way, particularly at the outset of meditation practice. But even then, after an hour of what seems like being pushed this way and that by body and mind, there is often an odd and surprisingly pleasant, joyful, and energetic feeling that arises. It is likely that in several tiny time spaces between effort and distraction there were moments of dropping away. The effort and distraction were never necessary, only the willingness to practice as it is. And through time, with practice, these moments grow, and a kind of self-enjoyment of mind and body emerges, and we "drop in" to our natural state. Zazen has been compared to the naturalness of a fish in water. The wavelike motion of a fish as it swims this way and that is like a mind and body that is not controlled, numbed, nor unconscious and automatic. It is playing freely, like a fish or a bird, clouds and water.

Having reached this quality of flow of body and mind, it is easy to become attached to the bliss, and to limit oneself to the pure enjoyment of body and mind at play. This is the "high" quality of samādhi, when our body and mind take on the color of the sky, the green of the trees. Yet there is a far deeper and richer possibility. The realization of body and mind dropped away is only the beginning. When we reach this place that is no-place, again and again, we launch ourselves into life itself. Or, as another Zen saying has it, when we reach the top of a hundred-foot pole, where do we go? We step out, and manifest our body in the ten directions. We let go. Completely, utterly, releasing our grip on even the bliss. And in that release, we find a wilder, open freedom, and responsibility. We meet our relationship with the world. We find we are the world and that there is plenty to do. From the high top of a pole we let go and see where we are, literally, right now.

Sitting on the subway, rickety-rackety sounds, the vibration in my butt, legs, feet. People sleeping, looking up, looking down, looking at me now, and zazen is not sitting or lying down, it is being alive and awake, inside and outside, here and now. Inside: the muscle of compassion, the muscle of steadiness, patience, kindness—it rests, calming fear and anger as they rise and fall. Outside: seeing that no matter what, hidden or revealed, there is kindness and love in each one of these fellow passengers.

When we first sit down to practice with our own body and mind, we might think that they are two. And we practice for a while and we recognize that body is mind and mind is body. And we start by thinking that we and the world are two. And we practice a while longer, and we realize that we and the world are one. And we practice a little longer, and we realize that we must act in the world, and that it is not a matter of one or two. It is just realizing our nature moment to moment, olive blossoms, mosquitoes, standing by a tree, a urine-stained alley. This is jumping off the pole.

Jumping off the pole offers us the possibility to practice for all beings. And while that might sound overly pious, it is in fact true. And somehow I don't think it matters whether we know it or not at the beginning of our spiritual path. Maybe we think we are doing it for our own well-being, our own salvation, our own happiness. How different is that from Mazu's doing it in order to attain Buddhahood? We may be mistaken as we enter the path, but as we move along, like Mazu, we are likely to encounter the real thing.

In an early Mahāyāna Sūtra, the *Vimalakīrti,* there is a wonderful scene in which the accomplished meditator Shariputra tells of what he learned about meditation from the great and worldly lay teacher Vimalakīrti. Shariputra is portrayed as austere and somewhat severe in his expression of meditation. We can imagine him sitting completely sealed in his concentration. One day Shariputra was sitting under a tree and Vimalakīrti came by and corrected him, saying true meditation is to appear in the activities of the ordinary people, not abandoning your samādhi and "yet showing yourself in the ceremonies of daily life."[11] What ceremonies of daily life? Those of the marketplace, the commons, the home. In Vimalakīrti's case, it was going to bars and brothels and talking with people. For many of us today, it is the ceremony of recycling the earth's resources, talking with an angry neighbor, mindful business practice, or as simple a ceremony as dipping your credit card with the samādhi of dropping away separation.

What is the ultimate most deep and profound realization? It is that we are not separate from markets and bars and subways and pollution and our responsibilities as integral beings in the world. Vimalakīrti is urging this holy man to see that we must let go of every shred of self-clinging, to drop off all notions of a separate self, all ideas of reality, of body or mind, let it all drop away. And what is left is the ceremony of daily life.

Consider how we approach these ceremonies of our daily life. The great Duke Ellington gave a wise teaching when he said, "It don't mean a thing if it ain't got that swing." It's true of music, of our meditation practice, of our lives. What is that swing? Isn't it the vitality, the presence, the spontaneity, the free improvisation of play? What meaning, what importance does our life have if it is missing "that swing"? When we encounter reality freshly, with full attention and nonseparation, we will naturally place the beat in the unexpected, yet perfect groove. We ourselves are in that groove and that is how we are able to swing. When we move out of the beat, out of the rhythm, we contract and get stuck again. And that stuck place hinders our ability to serve ourselves and others. Separating our understanding of body and mind, self and other, practice and fruition, we lose the beat and forget that we are all of these dualities. And when we let them drop away we become, as the Zen saying goes, like a dragon in water, a tiger in the mountains.

3

THE BROAD TONGUE OF THE TATHĀGATA

Spatial Breathing in Ch'an

MING QING SIFU
(DANIEL ODIER)

In the Ch'an tradition of Zaozhou, the emblematic master of the Tang Dynasty (618–907), we see how the spatial breathing sums up the entire Yoga practice. It is important to realize the practical way in which Ch'an differs from the Zen tradition as it is well known in Europe and America. Our tradition, based on the practices of the Tang Dynasty, emphasizes fluidity and spontaneity as opposed to the more ritual forms of the Japanese tradition.

The sitting position is different; we sit without rigidity, in a natural mood, warming and enveloping the base with a blanket to avoid tension in the joints. The waist stays in alignment; we don't push it back putting the spine in an angle, which tends to cut the flow of energy. We proceed by intuition more than by adopting a standardized posture. We recognize the capacity of the body to be a link between sky and earth and we let it resonate in the space, tuning it like a musical instrument. The hands are freely placed; they can touch or not, and the gaze is preferably open to the infinite space. The whole meditation process is about abandoning the limits of the physical body. All the senses are open and present. We don't shun the mind, we let it relax naturally and be one with the universe. Then samādhi will come naturally beyond any limits of the mind and body, which for the Chinese are not separate entities.

During more intense meditation sessions, we sit forty-five minutes and walk fifteen minutes and we repeat this process. The way we walk around the Buddha is not ritualized at all. We walk to relax, forming a great living maṇḍala around the spatial essence of the Buddha Mind. We walk freely, the arms following the movements of the legs, like we would when walking in the forest. The speed is free. Some walk faster, others slower. After a while, there is a sudden harmony developing spontaneously and we hear the soft sound of the robes pushing against the legs. At the sound of the percussion, we go back and sit again.

In the Chinese tradition, it is very important to avoid rejecting anything and to encounter the space with the whole being. We integrate art and beauty into the path, unlike the rather puritanical Indian Buddhism. Following the injunction of the *Avataṃsaka Sūtra,* we don't see the Buddha in one phenomenon, event, territory, nor way of being. We see the Buddha everywhere. Therefore there is not a single place, a single event, a single emotion that is not the Buddha. We see the Buddha everywhere without any separation. This power is great, and is a cardinal idea of the Chinese mind. It avoids any conflict with reality and is all-embracing.

The dharma is a teaching without an object. A stone, a river, a tree can expose the dharma as well as the infinite silence of our heart/mind. We are like the sky embracing the cosmos.

This premise is the key to the Yoga of breathing. We need a body that is totally connected to all levels of emotions and sensations and we allow our body to be infused by the space. We nurture life. We find joy without entanglements. The mind light is naturally profound and clear like a spring. We flow naturally. Zibo, a great Ch'an master of the sixteenth century, sums up this vision:

> With One Mind unborn, being and nothingness are not in opposition—even less so where there is a perceiver. Even so, once one mind is born, the six sense faculties are already provided. It is not possible to enter into enlightenment by abandoning these. . . . This being so, all things are the marks of the Tathāgata's broad tongue: sad songs, deep feelings, swearing and chiding, thorn forests and trees of beauty, gowns and caps, rites and music, drums and flute, drinking, eating, sex, right and wrong, good and evil, the clash of weapons, the formal dance, silent misty forests, noisy urban squares. Whether one has entry or does not, all depends on how one hears Buddha's tongue in every form.[1]

These practices and broad visions of the Path are the prelude to the great circulation of the breath. As long as we are not communicating deeply at all levels of the mind and body consciousness, we are limited and linked to our spiritual illusions, mistaking the form for the substance. In every path, there is a fatal virus which is the Path itself as we conceptualize it. This is a fatal trap that prevents the breath from flowing freely through space. The Chinese masters were not tender with students' concepts. They encouraged them to kill the Buddha. Some of them went as far as to physically destroy the images and statues of the Buddha. One of them used the wood of a Buddha statue to warm his cell during a terrible winter.

To liberate the breath, we have to abandon all our concepts and beliefs about the Path. This is the deepest Yoga. It makes us realize through samādhi and illumination that the infinite space of our heart is free of any form and is all forms at the same time. The breath, in a free space, will accomplish the absence of limits. The full cosmos will then inhabit our vast body. There is no other training for the Yoga of infinite breath than the abandonment of all our clinging, fixations, dreams, and illusions. We just have to empty the house, making it clear and shining for the breath to circulate and explode all the limitations of mind.

Then, as my Great Master Xu Yun (Empty Cloud) explained, "If, for one second, you have the experience of the unborn, the doors of the Dharma expounded by Buddha are useless."[2]

4

ZEN OR YOGA?

A Teacher Responds

SHOSAN VICTORIA AUSTIN

As I traveled home on an airplane recently, dressed in everyday robes, a passenger next to me asked me where I'd been. I said, "At a Yoga teachers' workshop."

"Really?" he asked, lifting an eyebrow. "Which do you practice—Zen or Yoga?"

As I'm an ordained Soto Zen priest who is also a certified Iyengar Yoga teacher, I answered, "Both."

"How can that possibly work?" he asked. The sounds of the airplane surrounded us as we hurtled through the sky. He told me he'd always thought of Buddhism as a religion like Christianity or Islam, and Yoga as a set of physical postures. "Christianity addresses the separation we feel between perfection and our life," he added. "What does Buddhism do? And what's spiritual about Yoga?"

My seatmate's very natural questions reflect a common view: that Yoga is practice for the body and Zen, practice for the mind.

According to Barbara Stoler Miller, a renowned scholar and translator, the notion that Yoga is only a body practice was born from a

Rāja Yoga presentation given by Swami Vivekanānda, a great teacher of Vedānta and Yoga, in Chicago in 1893. Later, though Hatha Yoga became known as a means of promoting health and balance, its role in mind training went largely unnoticed for up to a hundred years.[1]

The preconception that Zen and indeed all of the Buddhadharma (Buddhist teaching/way) is mind practice might be a Western reading of its traditional emphasis. The Buddha taught that all knowables come from mind. He did not add our cultural slant, which separates mind from body. Rather, he taught body and mind (nāma-rūpa) as one stage of a twelvefold chain of karmic causation culminating with birth, existence, and death.

I see the assumption of a mind-body split, Zen versus Yoga, as a feature of the English language, rather than as any actual separation between the territory of Buddhism and that of Yoga. Even attempts to integrate these disciplines may use language that reinforces this assumption. And then, these same assumptions are carried through into teaching, workshops, and books: for instance, among recent titles we find *Yoga Body, Buddha Mind* and *Zen Mind, Yoga Body.* These teachers and writers know both disciplines and are aware of the cultural judgments that surround them. Though experiencing the books and workshops would resolve the split, reading the titles alone would reify it.

Indeed, as my airplane companion noted, Buddhism is a religion, with all the forms of social, physical, and mental observance this word implies. Yoga is a path that unites our layers of experience. As B. K. S. Iyengar, the founder of the method I practice, has said, "Yoga is not a religion but a religious subject which enhances the religiousness of mankind."[2] Buddhism is a yogic religion; Yoga is not a form of Buddhism. Yet both Buddhism and Yoga cover much of the same ground—how to end suffering through orienting to one's true self (Yoga) or our true nature (Buddhism).

The yogic tools of Zen Buddhism include seated meditation (dhyāna), precepts (moral vows), study with a teacher, and everyday life. The main point of Zen is how to resolve suffering of body, speech, and mind through resting in three modes of reality: ultimate truth, conventional truth, and the skillful interplay between these two truths.

Yoga is a practical discipline that unites and silences one's whole being to rest in the Self (the capital-*S* Self, the eternal core of the soul, is distinguished from the transient small-*s* self). The process of studying precepts, postures, breath, and concentration harmonizes, then stills the waves of thought. Small self and big Self then act as one, with the fragrance of eternity.

My airplane seatmate's interest inspired me to newly consider some questions people have asked me for decades about my practice of Zen and Yoga.

I started practicing both disciplines in 1971, just after a near-death experience in a car accident. My first impulse (a premed math major, I was intensely focused on achievement) was to apply by rote my existing study methods to Zen practice. By the mid-seventies, when I moved into San Francisco Zen Center, I was spurring what I thought of as progress by forcing my legs into full lotus. In sesshins (meditation retreats), I would push to sit zazen all night. While these practices are not intrinsically harmful, in my novice's fervor I nearly burned out my nervous system in the first ten years of sitting. This is also how I began Iyengar Yoga. Because everything hurt, I felt I would damage myself further unless I could immediately address my issues. With priest ordination (1982) and dharma transmission (1999), I vowed to teach Zen in accordance with its yogic roots.

Before and since my teacher certification in 1988, I studied Yoga with senior Iyengar teacher Manouso Manos and others in the United States, and with the Iyengars in India. The Iyengars are among today's foremost practitioners of Patañjala Yoga—a group of interwoven, integrated disciplines, also known as Aṣṭāṅga Yoga (eight-limbs Yoga), outlined twenty-two hundred years ago by the person who codified Yoga, Patañjali. Deeper study and greater teaching responsibility sharpened my intention to be true to the method and to my teachers.

Initially Yoga allowed me to repair my knees, fix my back, and identify and address many of the obstacles that kept my seated posture from being meditative. These obstacles were physical, psychological, emotional, mental, and spiritual. By sticking with Yoga practice, I learned how to specifically identify and address the roots of suffering. I learned right effort. My experience became wide enough and deep enough to develop the near-death insights, and transcend them.

I was now orienting my practice toward personal, direct experience. Training in both Zen and Yoga entails setting the stage for certain experiences, observing the scene play out, and transcending the separation of player and played. What comes from each of these processes is the widened emotional life, intuition, and tools that we call wisdom. In both traditions, a teacher is one who directly experiences the truth through the forms of the practice, and who passes these ways of experiencing to students. But it is up to each student to transform the form of practice into direct experience.

Question: What is a beginner's direct experience like in Zen? In Yoga?

At San Francisco Zen Center, Saturday-morning practice begins with zazen instruction. A new student starts with a cup of tea and a brief tour. An instructor explains the bells and drums, and shows how to enter the meditation hall. The next step is to study the motivation and form of seated meditation posture.

Beginners learn the mechanics of sitting: leg positions, physical attitude of the torso, arm posture, Buddha's gaze. Thus "meditation" is practiced from day one.

By far the most common question comes from the beginner who enters the meditation hall expecting peace and quiet. As soon as the student sits down, thoughts and doubts arise: "Is this posture correct? Did I leave the stove on at home?"

This is completely normal. Habits and preconceptions of body, speech, and mind generally proceed like a stream. Starting to sit is like stopping midstream. Struggling to settle, one first feels the current's force and direction. At the same time, beneath the eyebrows, the beginner first meets that which is completely settled.

Meanwhile, at the door of a nonprofit or private studio, a different beginner enters an introductory Yoga class. The teacher directs the group to sit and chant "OM." The teacher demonstrates the first pose. When the student tries to copy that shape, he or she enters a new world. Exhilaration or despair balloons up and is witnessed: "I succeeded," "I failed." Repeating the pose, the teacher introduces an action: "Begin by putting all your weight in your heels." The pose begins to develop from the heels, from the student's foundation. Now bones and breath begin to support the pose. The student is discovering union.

Over the next few weeks, our Yoga beginner repeats the shape many times. The basic poses and actions become firm. A sense of direction begins to dawn—from the peripheral actions inward. At this point, the student is very concerned with physical movements and basic actions—with structure. This is bahiraṅga sādhana (external practice), the outer quest.

Question: What does Zen promise its students? And Yoga?

Life is suffering.

There is an origin of suffering.

There is an end to suffering.

The end to suffering is the Path.

Though these Four Noble Truths are Buddha's main teaching, they could just as easily be a summary of Patañjala Yoga. Both Zen and Yoga promise the practitioner a way to follow, toward the ultimate goal of ending suffering.

Buddha teaches that the root cause of suffering is thirst, conditioned by ignorance. Its remedy is the Eightfold Path of wisdom (right view, right intention), vow (right speech, right action, right livelihood), and contemplation (right effort, right mindfulness, and right concentration).

Patañjali teaches that suffering arises from identifying the seer (Self) with the seen (Nature), and its cure is their dissociation through the Eight Limbs of Yoga: the outer quest (universal morality, personal observance, āsana or physical postures), the inner quest (mastery of physiology and energy, involution, concentration), and the inmost quest (one-pointedness, transcendent union).

Question: How much of Zen is mind training?
As a form of Buddhism, Zen manifests the Eightfold Path. The word *Zen* is Japanese for the Chinese *Ch'an,* which transliterates the Sanskrit *dhyāna* (seated meditation). The essence of the path is that the yogic practice of Zen and its realization are one. Here is a taste of the essence of Zen from its founders in China and Japan:

> Buddha is Sanskrit for what you call aware, miraculously aware. Responding, perceiving, arching your brows, blinking your eyes, moving your hands and feet, it's all your miraculously aware nature. And this nature is the mind. And the mind is the Buddha. And the Buddha is the path. And the path is Zen. But the word Zen is one that remains a puzzle to both mortals and sages. Seeing your nature is Zen. Unless you see your nature, it's not Zen.[3]

> To study the Buddha Way is to study the self.
> To study the self is to forget the self.
> To forget the self is to be enlightened by all things.
> All traces of enlightenment drop away, and this traceless
> enlightenment continues forever.[4]

Suzuki Roshi, founder of San Francisco Zen Center, observed that practice is transmitted "warm hand to warm hand."[5] A teacher may use words, actions, or their opposite.

A few details of personal experience might be useful. Once responding to my question about practicing with the intolerable, my own transmission teacher, Sojun Mel Weitsman, in San Francisco, said, "Now, could you live in a way that is less horrible for you?" The resulting cleansing laughter allowed me to respond to the situation in an awake state.

Another time, Mel adjusted my use of the zagu (monastic bowing cloth) with his fingers every morning for eighty-nine days. On the ninetieth day, he said only, "Mmm." This is how the teaching has been transmitted from Buddha till today, with this attention to immediacy, to awareness, in the student.

From the outside, Buddhism looks ceremonial. It can be experienced as a formal tradition without inner meaning. But the meaning is there. With the transmission of monastic practice to the West, the form is refreshed. People are appreciating it anew, and this is transforming both the home culture and our own.

The transmission to each new country is colored by its culture. China incorporated Daoism, ancestors, and the work ethic; in Japan the arts and deep experiences such as wa (peace, group harmony), wabi-sabi (keen simplicity), kokoro (heart or deep feeling), and nemawashi (preparing the ground) developed with Zen. In America, we might contribute family practice, diversity, and mass media. But our cultural emphasis on physical objects and results could easily reduce the public perception of Zen to an art leading to mental skill. Business names such as "Zen Hairdressers," "The Zen of Investment," and "Presentation Zen" reinforce this interpretation of the term.

To understand how odd this is, substitute "Christianity," "Islam," or "Judaism" in the above titles.

One side of this new usage is that the term *Zen* signals skillful transformation. Another side is that using the term this way, without direct knowledge, caricatures it. Zen becomes impoverished as mere "mind training" without designating its vast field of experience.

Question: How much of Yoga is body training?

The eight limbs of Yoga have been transmitted in diverse traditions and styles. These include Hatha Yoga, usually understood as physical, Bhakti Yoga (devotion), and Rāja Yoga, understood like Zen as mind training leading to awakening.

Iyengar Yoga reinstates and revitalizes all three. B. K. S. Iyengar studied with Krishnamacharya, the South Indian sage who also taught Pattabhi Jois and Desikachar. Krishnamacharya studied with Ramamohana Brahmāchari. Ramamohana learned from the previous generation. However, B. K. S. Iyengar strongly innovated Yoga practice and teaching to include modern communication, the use of props, and the institution of group classes that many traditions use today.

In Iyengar Yoga, āsana (postures) and Rāja Yoga (so-called mind training) are not separate. Mind is not in the brain; mind permeates the whole. A beginning āsana practitioner copies shape and movement. As we cultivate external and internal alignment, we learn to experience layers of āsana as layers of mind. As perception and action unite, we directly experience the play of the elements, the energies of the body and Time itself flashing in Eternity. We know the nature of the universe through our own experience of self. We silently witness how the Divine expresses itself through us.

Though B. K. S. Iyengar is known for his precise teachings of alignment, his teaching of Patañjala Yoga does not end with the physical. About twenty years ago, I asked him once about a lump on my wrist. He responded that I had to learn to take the muscles evenly inward, so the bones would work. When I didn't understand, he asked me to hold out my arm and asked me how it was. When I couldn't tell, he held out his arm for me to touch. Wow. It felt completely at one—muscles, bones, everything doing the same thing. Suddenly I understood how "Yoga" means "union."

Question: How did Yoga become a word for a physical tradition?
B. K. S. Iyengar puts it succinctly:

> It is hard for the common man to grasp the intricacies of the traditional definition that Yoga is the process of stilling the consciousness and then merging the individual soul . . . with the Universal Soul . . . . [The average student] can be made to understand what Yoga is by exploring the concrete in him, the body . . . . Even today we tend to quarrel over the meaning and modes of Yoga . . . . One could assert that Yoga was merely physical,

> another, with equal authority, could assert that it was more mental and spiritual. A third person could label it as science or call it an art, education, religion, philosophy or even hocus pocus, without giving a thought to the development of man's total being.[6]

It can take many years to develop "peace in body and poise in the consciousness," as Iyengar phrases it, even with devoted practice. However, the shapes of āsana are relatively easy to learn, and physical practice offers a relatively quick feeling of well-being. Given America's cultural slant toward quick, painless results, is it any wonder that we have invented the thirty-day teacher-training course? Or that we mistake Yoga's physical forms for its meaning?

Question: But if Zen and Yoga both unite body and mind, aren't they really, in essence, the same path?
Yes and no. Though Zen and Yoga each define a Path toward ultimate truths about life, suffering, and the end of suffering, there are verbal, conceptual, and cultural differences along the way. These are too significant to ignore. In fact, these "along-the-way" experiences provide much of the grist for individual practice. They are the historical, communal foundation of each discipline and are nontransferable between disciplines.

For instance, while the Four Noble Truths could summarize both Zen and Yoga, the basic Buddhist vow, the Three Refuges, cannot:

> I take refuge in Buddha (own nature, awakening).
>
> I take refuge in Dharma (teaching, truth).
>
> I take refuge in Saṅgha (community of practitioners and all beings).

When the Three Refuges are taken in their literal sense, they become distinct from Yoga (or any other) practice. There are many such teachings unique to each tradition, and I read parts of the *Yoga Sūtra* and Buddhist texts as firewalls that may have been created specifically to preserve the individuality of each tradition in historical time.

That said, Yoga and Zen are both universal, too. They teach how to acknowledge and purify habits and conceptions; make body and mind still and one-pointed; and see a transcendent whole.

Question: Why would someone study both Zen and Yoga?

Physically, in Yoga āsana one generally assumes many postures, and in Zen meditation one generally sits, stands, or walks, but in both disciplines, seated meditation is key. The word āsana means "seat" or "posture" as well as "practice of postures."

Of Yoga's eight limbs (aṣṭāṅga), only one details āsana. The rest train an external and internal unity, concentration, and complete absorption (samādhi). Many people see āsana practice as a way of developing the equipment for meditation. But the experiences are fluid: you can see āsana as stabilization, and you can experience āsana as insight.

Zen is very simple. In the practice of Zen Buddhism, taking refuge in Buddha, Dharma, and Saṅgha provides the possibility of a sudden awakening to the truth. Going for refuge to Buddha, instead of elsewhere, is the basic act of a Zen practitioner. But what if your condition does not allow you to take refuge? What if you're having great difficulty sitting, or understanding how to proceed?

In this situation, I feel, adding a Yoga practice might be helpful. Yoga can search out obstacles of body and mind that otherwise may block the Zen practitioner from taking real refuge. One may find Yoga to be of help in removing assumptions or deadened areas blocking actual experience, thus creating a foundation for higher levels of consciousness. B. K. S. Iyengar says that people practice "meditation" in deluded or harmful ways, then beg him to fix them. Body and mind may come to insight, but the fruit of realization ripens only in firm ground.

On the other hand, Zen teachings of sitting, precepts, and work can be a revelation for the Yoga practitioner who has lost contact with any of the eight limbs of Yoga. The Buddhist refuges model how to dedicate Yoga practice to a wider view. Zen teachers remind students to rely on direct experience, and restore "what is known" to its rightful position of support. As losing the thread of direct experience in āsana can render it useless, even dangerous, a Yoga practitioner in a commercial community can benefit from living counterexamples. Meeting people who have vowed to maintain mindfulness and concentration can be of utmost use.

Equating Yoga with body, and Zen with mind, is a false duality. Any discipline that heals suffering must thoroughly address its causes in body and mind. Yet the words that communicate these practices are by nature limited. They automatically transmit omissions and differences in approach, based on the language's history and culture. Mainstream descriptions of Zen and Yoga include neither the Zen monk's long hours refining the āsana of zazen nor the yogi's experience of concentration in a supported pose.

No language can really touch the truth of either Zen or Yoga. Each is complete. And any practitioner who is specific, observant, responsible, willing, and respectful, can use help from the one, to reach an awakening in the other.

Question: How is Buddhism yogic?

Though people often speak of Buddhism as if it had arisen independently, Gautama Buddha's first step upon setting out to end suffering was to find a Yoga teacher. Alara Kālāma (Skt: Ārāḍa Kālāma) was a North Indian ascetic who emphasized direct experience. He taught the jhānas, yogic meditation states to quiet the discursive mind and realize insight into Nothingness. After penetrating Nothingness, Gautama did not feel that he had ended suffering. Nor did Alara Kālāma think that anyone could. So Gautama went in search of another Yoga master, Rāma, only to find that he had passed away.

Rāma's son, Uddaka, was teaching a very refined jhāna—Neither Perception nor Non-Perception. Attaining this, Gautama asked if Rāma had taught other methods. When Uddaka said no, Gautama resolved to transcend suffering on his own, through asceticism. This was a dead end. Self-denial required part of the mind to strive against another, creating war within the self.

Renouncing self-indulgence and self-denial, Gautama remembered a childhood experience of sitting under a tree, free from either extreme. This would be the key to his Yoga, the Middle Way. Sitting under the Bodhi tree, that night he reached the full awakening that he would transmit for the next forty-five years.

According to Barbara Stoler Miller, the Buddha's awakening occurred in a culture that had long been developing meditation practice:

> The *Yoga Sūtra* was certainly composed much later, but the elements that it shares with Buddhism may come from a common store of contemplative practice that was incorporated into Buddhism and developed there.[7]

In this context, she sees the Buddha's teaching as the first sustained expression and development of yogic ideas. Many core Yoga terms were created or influenced by the Buddha himself, or by later generations of practitioners:

> The important role of Buddhist technical terminology and concepts in the *Yoga Sūtra* suggests that Patañjali was aware of Buddhist ideas and wove them into his system. Two striking examples are the use of the term *nirodha* in the opening definition of Yoga as citta-vṛtti-nirodha, "cessation of the turnings of thought" (1.2), and the statement that "all is suffering (duḥkha) for the wise man" (2.15). Duḥkha and nirodha are crucial terms in the Buddhist doctrine of the Four Noble Truths, where they refer to the fact of universal suffering and to the means for the cessation of suffering, respectively.[8]

Generations of Buddhists in many lands developed forms that manifest this core, both in the meditation hall and in everyday life. For instance, the Soto Zen meal ceremony of Oryoki—"just enough"—embodies the Middle Way free from dualistic views of giver, receiver, and gift. If one substitutes "Buddha Nature" for "Brahmā," the main teaching of Oryoki could be taken straight from the *Bhagavad Gītā:*

> In the practice of seeing Brahmā everywhere as a form of sacrifice, Brahmā is the ladle (with which the oblation is poured into the fire etc.); Brahmā, again, is the oblation; Brahmā is the fire, Brahmā itself is the sacrificer, and so Brahmā itself constitutes the act of pouring the oblation into the fire. And finally Brahmā is the goal to be reached by him who is absorbed in Brahmā as the act of such sacrifice.[9]

Without explanation, the form invites a sense of unity that transcends suffering. Sitting in a maṇḍala with a meal offering at the center, and the abbots and teachers in the corner guardian positions, the meal begins with a sense of safety and harmony. This context is reinforced by invoking the names of awakened beings, and by reciting the Five Reflections (which also mirror the *Bhagavad Gītā*).[10]

- We reflect on the effort that brought us this food and consider how it comes to us.
- We reflect on our virtue and practice and whether we are worthy of this offering.
- We regard it as essential to keep the mind free from excesses such as greed.
- We regard this food as good medicine to sustain our life.
- For the sake of enlightenment, we now receive this food.[11]

The form is elaborate enough to include various levels of skill. Struggling to manage the basics of sitting, eating, and washing bowls, a beginner eats alongside a thirty-year practitioner, who might be absorbed in the nuances of handling utensils and cloths, and the subtle communication with the assembly in the meal hall. The real effort is not to be perfect, but to experience the interplay of oneness with the changes that occur during the meal.

In the particulars of the ceremony, we can see several different types of Yoga:

- Transcending the separation between self and other, by serving and receiving food as one: Bhakti, the Yoga of love.
- Cooking, serving, taking a role: Karma Yoga, the Yoga of action.
- Physical and energetic disciplines of breathing, bowing, chanting with the ears: Hatha, the Yoga of will.
- Insight into self, other, ultimate and relative truth: Jñāna, the Yoga of knowledge.
- Enthusiastically offering the food and studying oneself: Kriyā, the Yoga of purificatory skill.

Food eaten in this way carries the flavor of Yoga.

Question: What is an ongoing student's experience like in Zen? In Yoga?
An intermediate class has completed a series of strenuous poses, awakening and refining the student's body, energy, and perceptions. Now the teacher calls, "Śavāsana (Corpse pose)." Perhaps the student lies down and falls asleep. Perhaps the student experiences something completely new in his or her life—inviting the body to find complete rest, and the mind, complete presence. An intermediate teacher might choose the throat to be "the brain" of Śavāsana. How does the student find ease while meeting such an unfamiliar request? When his or her intelligence and physical effort withdraw to see, the body unites with the breath. Each inhalation and exhalation transmits a sense of self arising and dropping away, a glimmer of meditation. "Wow," the student might think. "What cool rhythms, my heartbeat, my breath, everything feels so harmonious, I feel great." Thinking mind has intruded, and the student must start again to create a state of alert repose.

Once the student is steady in āsana practice, the teacher may offer instruction in prāṇāyāma (vital energy training)—first in Śavāsana, later in a seated position. For prāṇāyāma to come to fruition in meditation and concentration, fulfilling the eight-limbed path, the student must have prepared the ground: mastery of all groups of āsana, plus Śavāsana and specific energy seals: Jālaṅdhara Bandha, Mahāmudrā, and Ṣanmukhi Mudrā.

The intermediate student has a thousand specific questions for the teacher:

- My knee is safe, but it is not yet completely balanced. What actions will satisfy my knee?
- My energy fluctuates in the pose. Please help.
- What āsanas might help me concentrate better in prāṇāyāma?
- What prāṇāyāmas should I practice?
- I seem to be controlling my breath unconsciously. How can I drop this habit?

As the basic poses become steady and comfortable, the student finds joy in deeper, subtler actions. He or she begins to notice how prāṇāyāma builds mental and emotional well-being. This initiates antaraṅga sādhana, the inner quest.

In the meantime, the continuing Zen student across town has been sitting and chanting every morning. As posture and intention stabilize, distractions become less compelling. Like the Yoga student, the Zen student is getting specific:

- Is my knee pain OK or harmful?
- How do I bring the stability of sitting into everyday life?
- The precepts seem to be naturally arising. Could you teach me about them?
- Is this job right livelihood for me or not?

The student might discover life issues that need attention or nourishment. This is a stage when I might recommend that the student take up an integrative, specific practice such as Yoga or tai chi.

Question: Is there a problem particular to an ongoing student of both Zen and Yoga?
One risk of an interdisciplinary approach is that with different types of input, the student may become confused. So I encourage the student to take one discipline as a main practice, and any other disciplines as support, for at least five years.

Question: If you practice both, how do you integrate the two practices?
Integration does not mean blending. In each I enjoy the fruits of the other, in physical, mental, and emotional conditioning, in learning how to detach from suffering, and how to experience things more purely. However, each form demands faithfulness. Zen transmission means I must hold the form as it has been transmitted to me. And an Iyengar Yoga teacher is someone who "teaches in the method set forth by B. K. S. Iyengar, without mixing in other styles of Yoga or other disciplines; and acknowledges the governing influence of the teaching of B. K. S. Iyengar on his or her practice and teaching of Yoga."[12]

Because of my responsibility to each discipline, it is crucial to my individual practice and teaching to keep them distinct. When we are seated in zazen, that is zazen. When we are doing Yoga, that is Yoga. If I blend the disciplines, I'm breaking my promise to respect the transmission of each.

My vow to teach Zen as a yogic school of Buddhist meditation requires the precise development of effort, which is exactly the substance of Hatha Yoga. Following Gautama Buddha's example, I have chosen to study with some of the finest Yoga teachers of our time. The practice of Yoga has matured my practice and teaching of Zen. And following the example of B. K. S. Iyengar, I faithfully practice my religious forms and exemplify them in my culture. Devotion to the truth of awakening, learned in Zen, informs and flavors my practice of Yoga. At a social, historical, and practical level, the disciplines are distinct; integration happens organically at the level of Self (the Yoga term) or Mind (the Zen term). Each of these disciplines compassionately assigns homework that transcends even the great teaching of its own form.

Question: How do you structure a practice that includes seated meditation and āsana?

My practice follows the seasons. In summer, I do prāṇāyāma early, then put on robes. After zazen and chanting, I do āsana. Often I do another practice later. This is the traditional order in Yoga—prāṇāyāma first, then meditation.

In winter, I often wake up an hour later. After zazen, I take a short break, then do prāṇāyāma. After tea, I may have time for āsana. If not, I practice later. Though this order is not traditional, it respects the later sunrise.

Once practice is accomplished, I take physical nourishment, then do the activities of the day. Before I sleep, I dedicate my practice.

Zen students studying Yoga as a support will schedule differently. Most beginners need only twenty to thirty minutes' āsana practice, three times a week, to experience the benefits of Yoga. Though many Zen students try to loosen up with āsana immediately before zazen, in my experience this is agitating, unless the body is very cold and dull. Best times for āsana are several hours after meals.

Yoga students sitting zazen as a support will also have special considerations. Most beginners who practice zazen five minutes at a time will find a first taste of Zen. Quiet sitting for five minutes at the end of prāṇāyāma works well. And if you are a Yoga student who does not yet practice prāṇāyāma, I suggest that you explore it before adding zazen.

Question: What do you do to not confuse them?

I use cues appropriate to each discipline. For instance, I wear shorts or tights and a T-shirt to teach Yoga, and robes or monastic work clothes to teach Zen. I stand in Zen or Yoga posture, and practice appropriate speech. When I teach āsana, I stick to the form "āsana class." In Zen, it's easier because of the Buddhist tradition of borrowing from the host culture. Faithfulness is my open question, an area to study during my home practice, and before I open my mouth to teach.

Question: May I validly enrich my teaching of one discipline with concepts from the other?
If you do so, you risk losing what makes each lineage a teaching. I suggest you first explore what your discipline teaches about the concept you feel needs enrichment. It may be more complete than you have judged. Though there are many overlaps, each discipline has its own logic and its own form. Each discipline brings the practitioner to ultimate truth and skill.

Study what each discipline uniquely teaches. Don't be afraid when the teachings present different paths to truth.

Question: How do I know on any given day whether to focus on seated Zen meditation or on Yoga?
When I requested ordination, my teacher was concerned that I might be a spiritual shopper. He asked that I stop attending Yoga classes. I immediately obeyed, and unintentionally ignored yogic self-study. In retrospect, this was a mistake, as I had so much to learn both from classes and home practice. The hiatus hurt my body and mind.

If a student is struggling with this type of question, I suggest that they ask both the outer and the inner teacher, and deeply consider the response. Make your decision a process of self-study rather than an event.

Question: What's the direct experience of an experienced student of Zen? Of Yoga?
The experienced practitioner of Zen or Yoga takes refuge in daily practice to refresh the fundamentals, nip obstacles in the bud, and renew his or her stability and ease.

The Iyengar student is practicing āsana at home as well as in class. Inversions are an everyday practice, and the student covers all types of poses regularly. The first pose of the day reveals the direction of that day's practice. Sometimes pain arises, as defenses drop and insights arise. Flashes of joy and integration arise. Mistakes trigger new efforts and insights. Poses begin to link with each other, and with the inner and outer self. Others begin to trust this student for advice.

The core and foundation of prāṇāyāma practice now is seated Ujjāyī. To close a prāṇāyāma practice, the student may sit silently meditating with head erect and hands in namaste, withdrawing the attention to its intimate, ultimate source. Sitting peacefully in accord with the rhythms of the universe and the Self, he or she is practicing antarātma sādhana (the innermost quest).

Meanwhile, the experienced Zen student sits zazen every morning. His or her everyday life unites practice and realization. A tiny event such as hearing a bell may trigger insight: how nothing is what we expect it to be (emptiness); how each thing is a miracle just as it is (form), and how emptiness and form inform each action (skill for the benefit of all beings).

Our Zen student might express his or her realization in a variety of ways: volunteering at a soup kitchen, practicing an art, just doing the dishes. To the outside observer, his or her practice may be completely invisible, highly visible, or just glimpsed.

Both the experienced Zen and Yoga student have a direct experience of some core concepts of each other's discipline. The Zen adept finds right action in standing, walking, sitting, or lying down. He or she can adjust the seated āsana with skill, and is continuously aware of energy and breath. The Yoga adept practices antarātma sādhana in any pose, and brings the fruits of Yoga to everyday life with friendliness, compassion, sympathetic joy, and equanimity.

Question: Which philosophy best describes reality?

Both the experienced Zen student and the Yoga student ask about Self or soul. Here a huge apparent contradiction arises between the two paths. Patañjala Yoga posits a unique essence of nature that does not change, and a self separate from consciousness (Sūtras IV. 14–17 and 23–26). Buddhism, however, does not posit or describe an independent soul or essence. Self is caused, and thus changes. Many philosophers assume that the Buddha denied the existence of self. However, this is not so.

Patañjala Yoga is based on Saṅkhyā philosophy, which is based on the dualism of puruṣa, Self, on one side, and prakṛti, Nature, on the other. Puruṣa is unconditioned and cannot act. Prakṛti, the play of Nature, is in constant activity and exists for the self to see its Self.

Buddhism is not usually thought of as dualistic. Ultimate reality and relative reality are not considered to be separate. They are ways of speaking about the same thing. Reality itself is not describable. All words are relative.

In my experience, the apparent conflicts between Zen and Yoga philosophy arise when we attempt to describe experiences beyond words. Direct experience of both "self" and "not-self" overflows their conceptual labels.

In practice, Soto Zen and Iyengar Yoga meet in refreshingly relevant and nourishing ways. For example, like Zen form, Iyengar Yoga āsana uses precise alignment to create an impossible task for the thinking mind.

So here is how my airplane seatmate and I ended our discussion. When a practitioner of Zen or Yoga applies effort specifically, checks action with perception moment after moment, and strives in a supremely intense way, he or she opens to the possibility of transcendence of small self.

As we watched the land come toward us from my companion's window, he and I agreed: the purpose of these kinds of practices is to live well. We both hope for no separation between universal light and our daily lives. Whether one is wearing monastic robes or Yoga clothing, the study of body and mind is the study of the self.

After we said goodbye and disembarked the plane, and I started home, I thought about the Halāsana (Plow pose) I would practice soon, to help me sleep. The next morning, at the sound of the bell, I would wake up, put on my robes, go to the meditation hall, and sit zazen. Both these disciplines are part of my everyday life. They both help me touch ground. And both are what I offer to the students I am honored to teach.

5

JOINING WITH NATURALNESS

ARI GOLDFIELD
AND ROSE TAYLOR

Yogic consciousness . . . arises from meditation . . . .
When the net of concepts is cleared away,
Genuine reality vividly appears.[1]

—DHARMAKIRTI, SEVENTH-CENTURY INDIAN BUDDHIST MASTER

Although the disturbing emotions, the five poisons,[2] may agitate your mind,
Look at their true face, and let them be self-liberated.
Whatever thoughts of despair may arise in you,
Know their true nature, and thereby gain courage.
When you know how to practice these points well,
You will be a relaxed yogini.[3]

—KHENPO TSÜLTRIM GYAMTSO RINPOCHE, CONTEMPORARY TIBETAN BUDDHIST MASTER

THE TRADITION OF Buddhist Yoga is vast and wonderful. It is profound in its insights that we can discover for our own and others' benefit, and rich in its variety of skillful methods that we can use to put it into practice. This chapter aims to present the key points of Buddhist Yoga[4] in a way that Buddhists and non-Buddhists alike will find helpful and applicable to their own practices of Yoga and meditation.

We will begin by looking at what the phrase "Buddhist Yoga" means, so that as we proceed to explore the practice of Buddhist Yoga, we will be well equipped with a clear understanding of what Buddhist Yoga is all about. Next, we will examine the three qualities of mental outlook that form Buddhist Yoga's foundation: renunciation, compassionate bodhicitta, and the profound view of the true nature of reality. At that point, we will be ready to learn how to apply the principles of Buddhist Yoga in physical exercise and dance. Then, we will see how we can practice Buddhist Yoga when our bodies are afflicted by illness, and learn why the great masters have taught that being sick is actually a more conducive condition for practice than being healthy. Finally, we will learn how to practice Buddhist Yoga in the activities of daily life, so that no matter where we are or what we are doing, we can live fully and joyously as yogis and yoginis.

What Does "Buddhist Yoga" Mean?

The words *Buddhist* and *Yoga,* and by extension the names for adherents of Yoga, male "yogis" and female "yoginis," can refer to such a wide range of meanings and images that it will be helpful to begin by looking at precisely what we understand these words to refer to.

Buddhist in Tibetan is "nang pa sang jeh pa." *Nang pa* literally means "insider," but not in the sense of someone in a club or group to which outsiders do not belong. Rather, it means "someone who looks inside"—someone who looks in at the true nature of things, particularly at the true nature of their mind. When we are not content to search for happiness or truth in outer objects or situations; when we recognize that there must be some deeper reality to the objects that appear to our senses and the thoughts and emotions that appear in our minds, this can be the beginning of our Buddhist journey to discover the true nature "inside" appearances and mind.

Sang jeh is the Tibetan term for "Buddha," and each syllable is a word with its own meaning. *Sang* means "awaken"—to awaken from ignorance of the true nature of reality into wisdom that realizes it. The true nature of reality—meaning the true nature of mind and all the phenomena it perceives—is luminous awareness. This awareness transcends conceptual labels and expressions, and even transcends the duality between the outer objects we perceive and our inner consciousness that perceives them. It is open, spacious, and relaxed.

Jeh means "expand," referring to how the qualities of enlightenment such as clarity, equanimity, love, compassion, and happiness all grow from having awakened into wisdom. In fact, these qualities are inherent within mind's true nature, and by training in Buddhist Yoga, our ability to actualize them grows and grows.

Thus, no matter what religious, spiritual, or philosophical tradition we may follow (or not), we act in harmony with Buddhist principles when we look beyond the surface of appearances, thoughts, and emotions into their true nature; train in awakening from ignorance into wisdom realizing this true nature; and train in engendering compassion and the other qualities of enlightenment.

"Yoga" in Tibetan is *nal-jor,* meaning "to join (*jor*) with naturalness (*nal-ma*), the true nature of reality." Yoga, therefore, is any and all of the practices by which we join with naturalness; by which we achieve our awakening into wisdom. And so although one might think that one could identify yogis and yoginis by the pure clothes they wear or the pure foods they eat, in fact anyone who dedicates themselves to practicing on the path of joining with naturalness is a yogini or a yogi. As the great Tibetan yogi Milarepa[5] explained:

> In my tradition, if you sincerely want to practice the Dharma, you do not have to change your name. Since you can reach buddhahood with a full head of hair, you do not have to cut it off, or change your clothes.[6]

How do we join with naturalness? To join with the naturalness of the outer material world, we must ascertain outer appearances' true nature, and rest within it. To join with the naturalness of mind, we must ascertain mind's true nature, and rest within it. Our bodies are the perfect place to focus on in order to do both of these kinds of Yoga, because as Milarepa taught, the body is the border where mind and matter meet each other. Our bodies are made of matter, yet matter that is suffused with mental sensation and feeling. Body and mind are interdependent: changes in the body affect the mind, and mind's perceptions and feelings bring about physical changes as well. By penetrating to the true nature of the body, we can discover the true nature of mind. And by ascertaining mind's true nature, we can discover what the body actually is. Ultimately, our practice of Buddhist Yoga reveals to us that the difference between body and mind is merely a conceptual one, and in the true nature of reality—nondual, inexpressible awareness—body and mind are inseparable.

This is why it is skillful to employ both body and mind on the path to enlightenment. If we were to focus too heavily on one or the other, our practice would be out of balance. The key, therefore, is to give appropriate attention to each, and to train in their interrelationship by involving mind when we work with body and involving body when we work with mind. Then our practice is balanced and whole, and we make good use of all available resources on our journey. We will begin to see how to do this in our next section on the three qualities of mind we develop in order to give our practice of Buddhist Yoga its soundest possible foundation.

Foundations of Buddhist Yoga

RENUNCIATION, BODHICITTA, AND THE VIEW OF THE TRUE NATURE OF REALITY

Renunciation can be a frightening word. In order to practice Buddhist Yoga, are we being told that we must renounce the people we love, the activities we enjoy, our work—our life as we have lived it?

The answer is no. Since Buddhism focuses on working with oneself from the inside out, rather than the outside in, its teachings do not command us to do anything. Rather, we are invited to investigate things for ourselves and to come to our own conclusion as to how to proceed, for that is the only way that our actions will be stable and confident.

What we are invited to explore in this instance is how happiness and suffering work. Our normal tendency is to try to find happiness in outer situations that we believe to truly exist: We view our bodies to be truly existent, and we want them to always be healthy; we view our friends and family to be truly existent, and we want them to always love us and treat us well; we view our livelihood to be truly existent, and we want to be financially secure now and into the future. Most of all, we think that our minds are truly existent, and so we want our minds to be happy and free of any agitation, worry, or anguish.

The problem is that we have very little if any control over any of these things, so when they manifest or change in ways that we do not like, we suffer. We suffer from bodily aging and sickness, from conflict in our relationships, from uncertainty and downturns with regard to our work and livelihood.

But this suffering only comes from clinging to ourselves and all these outer appearances as being truly existent. In this way, we suffer during the day for the same reason that we suffer in a dream when we do not know that we are dreaming. We may dream of getting physically sick or injured; of our friends and family doing hurtful things to us; or of having problems at work, and suffer in the dream the same way that we would during the day. But we do not suffer because these appearances are truly existent; we suffer only because we mistakenly believe them to be so.

When we look at our own experiences, we should ask ourselves, "Has believing in the true existence of my body, mind, friends, family, and work ever brought me lasting happiness? Or has it just made me vulnerable to suffering?" If through this examination, we gain certainty that there is no happiness to be found in clinging to these things as truly existent, that is authentic renunciation. It does not mean that we have to disregard or abandon our bodies, material things, or people themselves; only our clinging to them as being solid, truly existent entities. As the great Indian master Tilopa sang to his disciple Naropa:

> O son, appearances don't bind you, it's the clinging that
> binds you,
> So cut through the clinging, Naropa.[7]

When we cut through our clinging, and we interact with our bodies, people, and other things while we are informed by wisdom rather than ignorance, our relationships with them work much better and we are much happier. It is like a dream when we know we are dreaming—we do not cling to what appears to us as being truly existent, so our experiences of the world are open, spacious, and relaxed.

COMPASSIONATE BODHICITTA

The second quality cultivated by practitioners of Buddhist Yoga is bodhicitta,[8] the motivation to attain buddhahood for the benefit of all sentient beings. By attaining buddhahood ourselves, we will be able to help others reach the same level of full awakening, which will completely free them from suffering and bring them boundless happiness. The great masters have taught that bodhicitta is the most positive and powerful motivation we can have for our practice. As the Indian teacher Śāntideva proclaimed:

> If with kindly generosity
> One merely has the wish to soothe

The aching heads of other beings,
Such merit knows no bounds.

No need to speak, then, of the wish
To drive away the endless pain
Of each and every living being,
Bringing them unbounded excellence.[9]

The cause of bodhicitta is compassion, the wish that sentient beings be free from suffering. Compassion keeps our practice free of selfish purposes, gives it great energy, and keeps our minds open and spacious. And compassion is accessible to us all, because it is inherent in mind's true nature. Remembering this is important because it gives us confidence in our ability to be compassionate. We simply need to train in helping our naturally present compassion manifest.

The main way to develop compassion is to generate good feelings toward others. Firstly, we can bring to mind someone we are very fond of; we can recall how we enjoy being with them and the times when they have helped us. Then we should develop that natural friendliness toward those whom we have no particular feelings for; and then toward those people we have difficulties with and tend to view in a negative way.

The following verse, commonly recited in Tibetan Buddhism, is an excellent way to focus the mind in order to arouse these qualities of love and compassion for all beings:

May all beings have happiness and the causes of happiness,
May they be free from suffering and the causes of suffering,
May they always have genuine happiness that is untarnished by suffering,
And may they reside in great equanimity, free of attachment and anger toward anyone near or far.[10]

We also have good reason to be grateful to others, because it is in relation to them that we are able to develop our own good qualities of love, compassion, generosity, and patience. In the context of relating with others, we test the strength of our good qualities, and discover where we get stuck and need to work further.

Also, the more we learn about the true nature of reality, the more our compassion awakens and expands. For we discover that in genuine reality, nondual and luminous awareness, there is no difference between ourselves and others; there is no difference between the true nature of one being's mind and that of another. The true nature of mind of all beings is basically good. Whatever faults we and other sentient beings may appear to have, they are all temporary. As practitioners of Buddhist Yoga, we develop compassion for all beings that is grounded in our awareness of equality.

Opening Up from Narrow Self-Concern

OTHERS ARE AS IMPORTANT AS OURSELVES

When we train in compassion, we practice shifting our focus from narrow self-concern to considering the possibility that the happiness and suffering of others is as important as our own. Usually, unless it is expedient for us, we disregard the needs of others in our personal quest for satisfaction. So let us challenge that tendency.

If we imagine a world where we ourselves were completely happy, would we really consider it so perfect if those around us were suffering? Our happiness would be that much greater if everyone else were happy too. So when we have moments of joy, instead of selfishly guarding that feeling, we can share it with others by making the wish that all beings experience such happiness.

When we suffer, we have the opportunity to develop compassion by connecting with the suffering of others. For when we feel sad or despondent, we can think about how others have these feelings too. We can be willing to open up to the suffering of others. Sometimes in a moment of our own pain, if we try to help another person feel more uplifted—even with a simple gesture of friendship such as a smile or inquiry into their well-being—it can actually make us feel better too.

Great Compassion Is Unbiased

We do not do this only for close friends and family; in Buddhist Yoga compassion's scope is vast, which is why it is known as "great compassion." Ordinarily, we only have compassion for those whom we feel fond of and whom we feel are sympathetic and worthy of compassion, such as the victims of aggression. It is less often that we feel compassion for our enemies and people whom we dislike; whom we feel are unsympathetic, evil, or unworthy of compassion, such as the perpetrators of aggressive acts. However, that type of bias is not great compassion.

Great compassion includes friends and enemies, victims and aggressors in a completely equal way; it does not have any bias in terms of having more affection for one sentient being and less for another. To the extent that they do not realize their true nature, all beings suffer and are worthy of compassion. All beings have within them the completely pure, true nature of mind. So all beings—friends, enemies, victims, and aggressors—are equally worthy of compassion.

The Power of Compassion

In one Yoga class, after practicing Upward Bow, or Wheel, pose (Skt: ūrdhva dhanurāsana), we repeated the posture by first arousing a mind of compassion toward someone we wished to benefit. This simple technique enabled us to hold the posture longer, with more precision and energy. Mind's power really does increase when we harness it for a positive end.

In Buddhist Yoga, we are taught to arouse the mind of bodhicitta before every practice. This infuses our whole practice with compassion's power. And at the end of every practice, we dedicate its positive results to others. An example of such a dedication is the following verse from the *King of Aspiration Prayers*:

> May all beings throughout the ten directions, however many they may be,
> Always have happiness, be free from illness;

> May all beings be in harmony with the aims of the dharma,
> And achieve what they hope for.[11]

Dedicating the merit of our practice in this way is traditionally compared to pouring a glass of water into a great ocean. The fruits of our individual practice may seem small, but when dedicated to others, they join with a vast ocean of positive altruistic energy. Then the potency of our practice is never lost, and it benefits sentient beings until every single one attains enlightenment.

THE PROFOUND VIEW OF NONDUAL AWARENESS

The third quality of mind that Buddhist yogis and yoginis need is the view of the profound true nature of reality—nondual awareness. When we realize this true nature, our dualistic concepts and disturbing emotions dissolve, and we join with naturalness. The great yogis and yoginis describe that experience in countless beautiful ways, such as spacious, relaxed, luminous, blissful, and immutable. The Indian yogini Niguma sang:

> What throws you down into saṃsāra's deep ocean
> Are these thoughts of attachment and anger.
> But realize they don't truly exist,
> And all is an island of gold![12]

And the Tibetan master Khenpo Tsültrim Gyamtso Rinpoche sings:

> Look nakedly at these forms that are like rainbows,
> appearance-emptiness,
> Listen intently to these sounds that are like echoes,
> sound-emptiness,
> Look straight at the essence of mind—clarity-
> emptiness, inexpressible,

And fixation-free, at ease in your own nature, let go
and relax. Ahh, ahh, ahh.[13]

Stage One of Joining with Naturalness
THE SELFLESSNESS OF BODY AND MIND

To help us realize this profound true nature for ourselves, the Buddha taught us how to gain certainty about and meditate upon it in stages.[14] These stages help us to see the mistakes present in the way we ordinarily think about things, and how to rectify those mistakes with clearer understanding and experience. Along the way, our anxiety, confusion, and suffering diminish, and the spaciousness, clarity, and happiness naturally present within our minds emerge.

The first stage is to realize that in body and mind, there is no truly existent "self," no "I," no "me." All of our suffering comes from thoughts such as "I am angry," "I am sick," "I am hurt," "I am in pain." But all of these thoughts are predicated on the belief that there really is an "I" and "me," whereas in reality, there is not. The self that appears is therefore like a dream and an illusion, and this is the truth of selflessness.

We must gain certainty in selflessness through our own analysis of body and mind. Before analyzing, we each may think that we have one self, and that this self has a continuous existence from our birth to our death. But we must analyze: Where in body and mind is this single, continuously existing self to be found?

We may at times strongly identify the self with a part of the body; for example, when we have stomach pain and think "I am sick." But the body is not one thing; it is actually a multiplicity of parts. And none of these parts is permanent; they are constantly changing—constantly arising, dissolving, and replacing one another. So is any one of the multitude of these impermanent parts really "me"?

When we investigate mind, we find that it is not the self either. We have strong thoughts and emotional experiences that we identify as the self, such as when we think "I am afraid" or "I am upset." But we had experiences like that last year, too, which were replaced by other experiences, which were in turn replaced by yet other thoughts and emotions. Are any of the multiplicity of these constantly changing thoughts and emotions really "me"?

When we analyze, then, we find that the self only exists as the focus of the strong fixations of our concepts. Our thoughts are prone to fixating on one part of the body or one event in the mind and thinking, "That is me." But when we think like that, do we feel good? Usually, the stronger the thought of "me," the more tension, anger, and suffering we experience. In contrast, the more we can join with the naturalness of selflessness, the more relaxed, clear, and happy we are. We realize that the self that appears is like the self in a movie, in a lucid dream, in a magical illusion. The sense of separation and loneliness that accompany ego-clinging begins to dissolve, and that is wonderful. As the Tibetan yogi Kalu Rinpoche taught:

> If you wake up to . . . reality,
> You will know that you are nothing,
> And being nothing, you are everything.[15]

Stage Two of Joining with Naturalness

THE EMPTINESS OF BODY AND MIND

Body and mind are not only of the nature of selflessness, they are also of the nature of emptiness. "Emptiness"—which the Buddha taught is the true nature of all phenomena—means that whatever phenomenon appears to our senses or thoughts, it does not truly exist as what it appears to be. It is a mere appearance, like an appearance in a dream or an illusion, and its true nature is beyond duality, beyond concept and expression.

Emptiness is too profound for most of us to be able to immediately grasp. However, if we approach it in a step-by-step way, we can understand it, gain certainty in it, and experience it, in the same way that the great yogis and yoginis do themselves.

Let us begin this gradual approach into emptiness by analyzing the body. We have a conceptual idea of the body, but when we try to actually find the body, we cannot, because "body" is just a label, a name given to a collection of smaller parts. If you try to identify your body by pointing to it, you cannot do so. When you point, your finger may touch your head, chest, an arm, or a leg, but never an entity called "body." The same is true when you try to point to an arm—you can point to the upper arm, lower arm, or hand, but "arm" itself is also just a name given to a collection of smaller parts. This is true down to the subtle particles that constitute the body—they are merely names given to collections of smaller parts, and even the tiniest of them cannot be found to be anything more than merely a name. Therefore, the body is not actually made of any substance that can be found under analysis. The body is empty of matter, so its true nature is emptiness, and its appearance is like a rainbow or a body of pure light. As Milarepa sang,

> My body is appearance-emptiness, like a
>   rainbow in the sky.
> It cannot be identified, so my attachment to
>   it has dissolved.[16]

Mind's nature is also emptiness, because in essence it is inexpressible and inconceivable. For example, if you eat a piece of fine chocolate, you have a mental experience that you cannot convey in words. You may describe it as "sweet," or "delicious," but if you are asked, "What is sweet like? What is delicious like?" you quickly run out of words that can describe your experience. The same is true for even the strongest emotions. If you have the feeling "I am angry," but then you go past the label "anger" into the experience itself, you discover that no words can actually describe it.

The same is true for happiness, sadness, calm, worry, pleasure, and pain—all the labels we superimpose on mind cannot actually describe mind's unchanging, inexpressible nature. And when we go past those labels and rest in that inexpressible nature of mind, we experience the Dharma-kāya, the enlightened mind of the Buddha that is our own mind's true nature, and the clarity, bliss, and emptiness that are inseparable from it. As Milarepa sang,

> All thoughts are free in being Dharma-kāya,
> It's awareness, clarity, and bliss,
> So to meditate, rest uncontrived.[17]

Body and Mind's Ultimate Nature

The ultimate naturalness of body and mind is that they are inseparable. As the Indian yogi Dombe Heruka sang,

> Body and mind—nonduality,
> Spacious and relaxed transparency.[18]

The body, free of self, free of particles of matter, is the dance and play of mind's native luminosity. The experience of joining with this naturalness is like dancing in a dream when you know you are dreaming! Dualistic thoughts dissolve; and nondual awareness, luminous and blissful, manifests. This is the fruition of Buddhist Yoga.

Buddhist Yogic Exercise

One of the methods to realize the fruition of Buddhist Yoga is yogic exercise. While there are many forms of yogic exercise, this presentation is based on teachings given by Khenpo Tsültrim Gyamtso Rinpoche. In Khenpo Rinpoche's system, the actual exercises are best learned under the direct guidance of an instructor, but the key points on how to work with the body and mind can be applied to all kinds of movement.

In yogic exercise, we have the opportunity to work with the mind and body in motion but still within the context of a formal practice. It may initially be more challenging for us to meditate while moving, but movement also helps dispel mind's dullness and agitation, two of the main obstacles in meditation. In this way, movement can be an excellent support for meditation.

Also, because we are continually moving in our daily lives, yogic exercise helps us develop the ability to bring that practice mind into our daily activities. We learn how to join with naturalness in all life circumstances, up to and including the point of death.

INTENTION

RENUNCIATION, BODHICITTA, VIEW

Recalling a Buddhist Yoga practitioner's three qualities of mind guides our intention when we practice yogic exercise. First, while exercise may beautify our bodies, enhance their health, and lengthen our lives, we renounce clinging to the body as truly existent. Whatever the body's condition, it cannot provide lasting happiness. Ultimately, the body is unreliable; however we try to preserve it, most of us will experience sickness and the gradual aging of the body, and all of us will finally relinquish the body in death. So, we are motivated to practice in order to help ourselves relinquish our clinging to the body and to realize its true nature.

Second, we generate the mind of bodhicitta. The aim of all Buddhist Yoga practices is not merely to benefit ourselves but to benefit all beings. So we begin our practice by making the wish that all beings be free of ordinary sickness and suffering, and also free of the ultimate sickness of clinging to the self and appearances as truly existent; that they too join with naturalness.

Finally, we practice with the motivation to realize the truth of the view, as succinctly expressed by Khenpo Rinpoche in the following verse:

> The nature of the body is appearance-emptiness, like a rainbow.
> The nature of the mind is luminosity-emptiness, like a water-moon.[19]

The nature of feelings is bliss-emptiness, inexpressible.
While remembering these three views,
Move and move while resting in the unmoving state.[20]

THE KEY POINTS OF YOGIC EXERCISE

The most profound way to apply the mind during any activity is to focus on the true nature of reality. The mind's true nature, nondual awareness, the union of luminosity-emptiness, is like a vast ocean in which thoughts and feelings are like waves inseparable from that nature. Therefore, we do not need to reject or subdue thoughts; we can let them naturally dissolve back into luminous awareness, just as waves dissolve back into the ocean. Simply rest the mind in luminosity-emptiness; when a thought arises, look directly at its essence, and relax in its true nature, luminosity-emptiness.

This is an excellent method for helping us release our habitual thought patterns, so that we can join with the naturalness of the way things actually are. But we also have a variety of other techniques to help us do this while specifically working with the body in yogic exercise.

At the beginning of the exercise session, mentally focus on the energy point four finger widths below the navel, deep in the center of the body. By focusing on this point, prāṇa (the subtle energy in the body) and mind gather there in the body's core, rather than being scattered in many directions. This clarifies one's practice and makes it effortlessly energetic.

Try to maintain awareness on this point throughout the session. It is fine to move your attention to other parts of the body, but also maintain some connection with this point as the source of movement and awareness.

When moving, whether slowly or quickly, generate internal vigor and strength. Move in a relaxed and natural way, but let your movements have inner strength coming from the central core of the body. Moving in this way energizes our practice, brings clarity to the mind, and helps protect us from physical injury.

In actual fact, the body is constantly moving—every part of the body is in constant motion, changing all the time. In its coarse state, the cells of the body are always moving back and forth; and in the subtle state, prāṇa is always moving through the nāḍīs (subtle channels).

While we move our bodies in exercise, we can feel that we are joining our external motion with our body's continual internal movement. So rather than revving something up and struggling to move the body, just relax and join the body's natural flow of movement.

By joining with the body's natural movement and energy in this way, we can transcend our notions of tiredness and lethargy. There is no place such tiredness can actually be located because the body's atoms themselves do not have the thought of being tired, and those atoms do not even truly exist.

This is the main point to remember about the body: it is not truly existent. We recall our certainty that this body is not made of matter; it is appearance-emptiness like a rainbow; it is purely the energy and play of luminosity-emptiness, like a body in a dream when we know we are dreaming. Then as we move, instead of feeling we are heaving around a body of muscle, bones, and blood, the body feels naturally light and luminous.

Not only are our own bodies appearance-emptiness; so are the bodies of others, as well as the surrounding environment. Neither our own bodies nor any of the outer appearances we perceive are made of the tiniest atoms, so no dividing line between these objects actually exists. As you move your body, dissolve fixation on the duality of your own body here and the surrounding environment out there; melt into space.

As we dissolve our reference points in this way, we also challenge our habitual views of spatial location. Ordinarily, we think we are on the top of the planet, right-side up. But directions as well are dualistic concepts that do not truly exist in nondual awareness.

This can be particularly useful to remember when we do inverted postures. Such postures can be very challenging, in part because we are so attached to looking at the world right-side up. In inversions, seeing the world in such a different way can make us disoriented and nauseous.

But when we work with dissolving our attachment to the concepts of direction, we find that inverted postures feel increasingly comfortable and natural.

We can work like this with dimensionality as well, and transcend the dualistic concepts of big and small. As described in the *Vimalakīrti Sūtra,* highly advanced practitioners who directly realize the true nature of reality are able to place a great mountain inside a mustard seed without decreasing the size of the mountain or increasing the size of the seed. As you move, dissolve your notions of size. Increase the size of your body so that it feels like a mountain filling space. Then decrease it so that it feels like a grain of sand in the vastness of space.

As we soften our dualistic concepts—matter and mind, self and other, up and down, big and small—the body and the environment reveal a gentler quality. Experience is much softer than when we are clinging to ourselves, objects, and ideas with heavy conceptuality. This is because we are closer to experiencing things as they actually are. Our experience is like waves on the ocean of nondual awareness, luminosity-emptiness. We dive into the ocean, relax, and move within the waves of luminosity. This is joining with naturalness.

How to Use Sickness to Enhance the Practice of Buddhist Yoga

The view of Buddhist Yoga is that sickness is our friend. It benefits our practice even more than being healthy does.

How is that the case? In general, when things are going well for us—when we are healthy, materially well off, surrounded by loving friends and family—it is easy to let all of these alluring appearances distract us from our practice. In contrast, when we suffer, we naturally have a strong incentive to free ourselves from clinging to our suffering as being truly existent, and to find its true nature—nondual awareness, spacious, luminous, and blissful. This is why Milarepa sang, "Adversity has been very kind to me."[21] His life's difficulties spurred him to realize that "the suffering being bliss feels so good that feeling bad feels good."[22]

The renowned Tibetan yogi Gyalwa Gotsangpa[23] endured severe and lengthy illnesses, among them an imbalance of wind-energy that produces symptoms similar to what modern medicine calls anxiety disorder. But Gotsangpa persevered with meditating on the true nature of his illness, and he achieved profound realization as a result. He sang many songs about how to take illness to the yogic path. One verse from such a song is:

> The illness and its painfulness have neither base nor root
> Relax into it, fresh and uncontrived
> Revealing Dharma-kāya way beyond all speech and thought
> Don't shun them, pain and illness are basically good.[24]

We can learn how to practice Gotsangpa's method by studying the meaning of this verse. The first line describes how illness and the suffering it causes us do not truly exist. How can we know that sickness is not real? Because, as Gotsangpa sings, it has no basis where it exists, no root or origin where it comes from. If we look in the body, we do not find sickness; we find cells that are made of atoms, atoms that are made of smaller particles, which are in turn made of even smaller particles—we cannot find even the tiniest particle of matter in the body. There is no root or basis for sickness in a body that is not actually made of any particles of matter.

And if we look in the mind, we do not find sickness there either. We may find a thought "I am sick," or "I am in pain," but if we ask ourselves, "What is that experience of sickness and pain actually like?" we quickly run out of words to describe it. So we find no sickness in the mind, only the inexpressible and luminous awareness that is the true nature of all thoughts and emotions.

Therefore, suffering from illness occurs only from the mistaken belief that we truly exist and our sickness truly exists. It is like being sick in a dream. The sick body that appears in the dream is not made of any particles of matter, so it is not really sick; and the dream thoughts of being sick do not truly exist either. If we do not know we are dreaming, however, we think the sickness is real and we suffer from it. But if we know we are dreaming, we know that the sickness is a mere appearance that is not real, and it does not cause us any suffering at all.

Once we know that the sickness does not truly exist, what should we do? Simply relax into its basic nature. We do not need to try to make it go away, make it improve, struggle with it in any way, or change anything at all. When we relax uncontrived like this, our experience of sickness's basic nature is always fresh, new, and luminous. In fact, it is nothing other than the enlightened essence of mind, Dharma-kāya beyond thought and expression. Therefore, there is no reason to shun pain or illness, because they are basically good.

When we are sick, it is helpful to sing Gotsangpa's verse, to meditate on its meaning, and to think, "This is like being sick in a dream when I know I am dreaming." Think of your body, particularly the part that is sick, as being appearance-emptiness, free of particles of matter, perfectly pure, like a dream body or a rainbow. Let your mind relax in its own basic nature, inexpressible awareness.

While sustaining this view and meditation, do some easy exercise with the sick part of your body if you are able to. Just to move that part of your body even in a subtle way is beneficial. If you cannot physically move, focusing your mind on the sick part of your body and feeling its natural movement is sufficient. The Tibetan masters teach a special skillful method here: When you exercise, think of the sick part of your body as being pure space. So if you have stomach problems, you visualize that where your stomach normally appears, there is just empty space. This is a powerful method that is very good at reversing the strong clinging we have to the sick part of our body as being truly existent.

When we use these methods, sickness enhances our practice of joining with naturalness, and we learn how sickness is not our enemy, but rather, one of our kindest friends. We can sing, as Gotsangpa did on another occasion:

> My sickness is not a problem—
> It clears away what obscures my mind,

Gives birth to the greatest qualities,
And enhances my realization.
So being sick fills me with joy![25]

Practice in Daily Life

Going, wandering, sleeping, resting—I look at mind
This is virtuous practice without sessions or breaks.[26]

—Milarepa

Modern life can be so fast-paced, busy, and demanding that it is easy for us to feel like we do not have enough time to meditate. However, Buddhist Yoga is actually ideally suited to being practiced right within our daily activities. By briefly reflecting on renunciation, bodhicitta, and the profound view from time to time during the day, we blend practice and daily life together. We train in acting without attachment, with compassion and bodhicitta, and with certainty in the true nature of whatever is happening. This allows practice to flow continually, without being confined to meditation sessions and breaks.

The only obstacle to joining with the naturalness of the appearances of daily life is fixating on them as being truly existent. The more we fixate on something, the further we separate ourselves from its true nature, and the more narrow-minded and agitated we become. To help us counteract that tendency, the Buddha taught the practice of the "illusion-like samādhi"[27] in verses like this one from *The Sūtra of the Noble Collection:*

All the images conjured up by a magician,
The horses, elephants, and chariots in his illusion,
Whatever may appear there, know that none of it is real,
And it's just like that with everything there is.[28]

Khenpo Rinpoche revised the first two lines to make them more applicable for modern practitioners:

All the images conjured up by a director,
The cities, cars, and airplanes, everything that's in the movies,
Whatever may appear there, know that none of it is real,
And it's just like that with everything there is.

Khenpo Rinpoche regularly sings verses like this one as he goes about his daily life, and frequently composes his own spontaneous verses as well, such as this one that he sang while swimming in the ocean:

In this illusory ocean,
A dreamlike person,
Swims like a water-moon,
And crosses over into equality's expanse.[29]

We can adapt this verse for all the different activities we undertake. For example,

In this illusory grocery store,
A dreamlike person,
Stands in line like in a movie,
And crosses over into equality's expanse.

Equality's expanse is the true nature of reality, nondual luminous awareness, in which dualistic differences, distinctions, and contradictions do not truly exist. All such differences are equally dreamlike and illusory—appearance-emptiness—and we cross over into equality's expanse when we see this.

Even the activities that we consider spiritual and those we consider mundane are equality, and every moment of mind is an opportunity to remember equality and join again with naturalness. By doing so we are not creating an alternative version of reality or just making things up; rather we are dropping our conceptual habits that obscure naturalness. As the Tibetan master Chögyam Trungpa explains, "The universe is constantly trying to reach us to say something or teach something."[30] We are always invited to reconnect with naturalness; we just need to accept the invitation.

Conclusion

In practicing Buddhist Yoga, we join with naturalness by relinquishing the burden of attachment; developing great compassion; and meditating in nondual, luminous awareness, the true nature of reality. Through applying these methods in all phases of our activity, our experience becomes open, spacious, and relaxed. Initially, we have to apply more effort, but gradually we experience the benefit of this approach to life, and practice becomes natural and joyful. When we do not fixate on situations as truly existent, all circumstances become workable. Fear and self-doubt fall away, and our ability to benefit ourselves and others grows.

6

ZEN BODY

EIDO SHIMANO ROSHI

As far as we know, Śākyamuni Buddha, before beginning his ascetic practice, was trained in Yoga and in sports and was very fit. Nevertheless, his mind was not at peace. His easy and comfortable upbringing did not draw him any closer to understanding the roots of life and death, or the cause of duḥkha (suffering). After leaving the five ascetics who were his practice companions, he started to thoroughly investigate the relation between body and mind, health and peace, and he systematically dropped what went against peace and cultivated what could increase it. He had gone to the end of what a human being can endure, and realizing he was not coming closer to his goal, he accepted an offering of rice cooked in milk and proceeded to abandon his former ascetic practice. He clearly realized that the body is as indispensable as the mind for finding ultimate liberation.

In modern Western civilization, religion has been regrettably reduced to intellectual study. The physical aspect of Judeo-Christian practice has been almost relinquished. While Buddhism was originally a religion of perfect body-mind integration, nowadays, even in Oriental countries, it is fading in favor of ritual and organized events. After the Industrial Revolution in England, life became more and more comfortable, and human beings were less and less allowed to use their own bodies. As a result, body and mind became disconnected from each other. This is where real dualistic ways of thinking began. Human beings started to overestimate their brain and neglect the hidden power and intelligence of the body.

Yet, modern people are not satisfied with mere study and literature, and the body gets diseased when not used properly. The Buddha's Four Noble Truths are timeless and are vividly experienced by modern people as well, namely, (1) life is suffering; (2) cause of suffering; (3) there is an end of suffering through the practice of (4) the Noble Eightfold Path. The last point of the Noble Eightfold Path discovered by the Buddha under the bodhi tree is right meditation. In order to meditate, we need our body. We also need our breath, which is of vital importance, to say the least. From the day we were born, we have been breathing freely, without the need to be instructed. Upon reaching adult age, filled with knowledge and concepts, the breath not being cultivated becomes shallow and short. Impatience, anxieties, short temper, lack of confidence, instability, and even stomach ulcers and high blood pressure, all come from the breath not being allowed to flow freely. In Zen Buddhist training, three things are really essential: (1) regulated breath, flowing in a (2) healthy body, and a (3) healthy mind (in this case, psychological mind) with a quest. Those three essentials flow into one when the spiritual aspirant is healthy.

The reason Buddhism and meditation are gaining interest in the West is that it addresses this particular problem and offers a practical solution. Many of my students come from a Judeo-Christian background, and though their philosophical and religious (academic) knowledge is plentiful, they don't feel satisfied. Unless we truly return to the source of our original nature, which is our birthright, our innate wisdom before knowledge took place, we cannot rest at peace.

In Zen Buddhism, sōji (cleaning) is of extreme importance. Not using any appliance, but using bamboo brooms and wet rags, the body is highly stimulated. This stimulation influences our breath, and therefore our state of mind becomes more clear and present. Chanting sūtras in a loud and enthusiastic voice has the same effect.

The Sino-Japanese word for "practice" is *shu-gyō*. *Shu* is usually translated as "training," *gyō* as "action." Very casually, people translate it as "ascetic discipline." But I would like to emphasize the action in body, mind, and thought. Without action, we cannot pursue any practice or discipline. Without mind, we cannot be thoughtful. Without thought, we cannot even be attentive, not to speak of questioning essential matters (who is it who is doing shugyō?)

All those who have a quest for truth must realize once again that body and mind are inseparable. Followers of the way must not forget how essential the body is in order to carry on their practice.

In *Shōbōgenzō (Shinjin Gakudō*—Studying the Way with Body and Mind) Master Dōgen said the following,

> To study the way with the body means to study the way with your own body. It is the study of the way using this lump of red flesh. The body comes from the study of the way. Whatever that may be which comes forth from the study of the way is the body. The entire world in the ten directions is nothing but the true human body. Life, death, coming and going are the true human body. Using this body we relinquish the ten evil deeds and keep the eight precepts, thus taking refuge in the Three Treasures and leaving home.[1]

7

MIND AND BODY AT EASE

SARAH POWERS

HATHA YOGA IS an introspective path of self-transformation that utilizes the body as a vehicle for harmonizing and strengthening one's energy. With balanced energy, we are better able to understand and free our minds, as well as develop an open and receptive heart. Mindfulness is a meditative awareness practice that develops a capacity to attend to our body, emotions, mind, and the environment with a receptive, noninvasive attitude. When we braid Hatha Yoga and mindfulness together as our practice life, we create a potent opportunity to diminish the suffering that is fueled by our habits of distraction and aggression as well as to increase our happiness as we begin to enliven our natural vitality and discover our authentic nature, an alert quality of presence and openness.

Physical Yoga practices involve placing our bodies in various shapes and, while focusing on the breath, directing our attention to specific areas within us as we alternate holding and flowing from pose to pose. This kind of practice not only strengthens the bones, muscles, and systems of the body but develops what I will call active attention. We learn in a nondistracted way to increase the potential for greater vitality within and between the body and mind. The attitude we foster is directive and is a main feature of our discerning intellect that develops as our practice continues. There is an additional aspect of our intelligence that similarly requires alert interest, yet instead of altering the body or mind, requires that we simply observe these qualities without interfering in their flow in any way. This kind of training can be called receptive attention and is what we develop in mindfulness practice. Practiced together, we develop the capacity to be both active and receptive while on the mat, as well as in our life.

I have found it very helpful to develop these complementary Yin and Yang qualities of attention in distinctively active and receptive postural practices. While I do engage in receptive attention in active practice and active attention in a receptive practice, a slow flow or Yang-style practice can be an appropriate style to heighten our responsive attention, while a Yin floor practice that holds poses for longer periods creates a natural container for receptive attention. Since so many Yoga classes already focus on the directive features of attention to the body and mind, I have felt inspired the last few years to focus on the receptive ones, not because they are better but because they require skillful guidance, as they are harder to develop and are often less popular in many Yoga classes. I have found the insights that can arise when we rest in a receptive attitude open us to deeper truths about ourselves that can directly enhance the way we operate in daily life. If our practice includes a receptive element and is genuine and skillful, we should notice direct shifts in how we relate to challenging circumstances in ordinary moments, feeling better able to connect with ourselves with increased care and kindness, while feeling more able to meet unavoidably difficult circumstances in life without adding suffering to our suffering.

In order to develop this attitude of sensitive, nonmanipulative attention, we need a simple and quiet āsana practice in order to discover what's going on in our body moment to moment, to learn to tolerate difficult sensations while opening to a wide array of emotions, all the while attempting to stay intimately connected to our experience in this body.

When we are in a pose feeling challenging sensations pulsing through us, our resistance to difficult sensations can cause even more suffering than the pain itself. This insight into how we add to our suffering when we struggle, and how awareness of the resistance can diminish the suffering, develops a practical skill we can apply to simple moments outside practice.

Last night for example, I was lying on my bed bathed in sweat from the searing heat. At a certain point the ordinary discomfort turned into blazing hot flashes across my entire body. Everywhere was running water; my forehead, my neck, my legs. . . . Lying there, I became utterly intolerant of my experience and before I knew it, I was defiantly standing, almost expecting I would encounter an enemy lurking. As if catching myself in the mirror, I stopped and looked at what was happening inside me—the raging heat as well as the familiarity of discontent. As my attention dropped down and in, I simply felt the firm ground under my feet, sticky sweat pouring down my belly, and the heavy warm air all around me. Without planning it, I dropped into awareness of sensations, the First Foundation of Mindfulness.

As I simply watched all this, I became aware that my angst had effortlessly slipped away and I was now feeling calm and present. I erupted in laughter at my familiar response to discomfort. Again and again I am astonished at how a forceful and indignant emotion can simply decompose as my attention turns toward my direct experience mindfully. I lay back down noticing that the next moment was no less fiery, yet my inner attitude had shifted. My experience of the sweltering heat had changed simply because my attention had shifted from resistance to observation.

Mindfulness practice is a method that helps us pause in the midst of any experience we are struggling with, helping to relieve many moments of ordinary suffering in our life. This practice has helped me become increasingly interested in not only listening to the inner messages I tell myself while in a pose, or while meditating, but also paying attention to my self-talk throughout the day. A popular internal and mental line I have caught myself saying is, "I can't stand this another moment." It might occur in the middle of a difficult hip-opening Yoga pose, during an uncomfortable meditation session, or in the middle of an argument with my husband. When I am able to interrupt my struggle with what's happening long enough to question my contracting attitude, I can ask myself, "Where am I not able to stand this another moment?" Then I go on a search: "What's going on in my body right now?" This is the First Foundation of Mindfulness, mindfulness of the body.

In order to entrain this capacity to simply observe our raw and direct experience without being seduced into believing in any commentary, we need to create a safe, optimal environment for reestablishing a renewed curiosity about learning how to be with ourselves in difficult moments. Our Yoga sessions are an optimal place for developing this quality of sensitivity toward our inner world. As we settle into a pose, we might be experiencing some tension in the abdomen, or some blockage in the shoulder. When we observe with a mindful attitude, our query becomes threefold: "What's my current situation?" (knowing what's happening now), "How does this feel?" (investigating the particular sensations dominating the moment), and "What's my attitude toward this sensation?" (paying attention to how I am relating to what's happening, while turning back to the direct sensation occurring now). We segregate these three features, learning to disentangle the direct body sensations from the mental factors, garnering insight into how both pleasant and unpleasant sensations are inevitable and how our mind states determine whether we suffer or not.

Giving ourselves time each day in a receptive practice such as Yin Yoga to inhabit our bodies in a nonstriving way creates an optimum environment for developing mindful attention toward the body. In the beginning of mindfulness practice, we track what is arising in us moment to moment without acting out for or against what we notice. This is sometimes called bare attention and allows us to observe the distinction between sensations in the body and attitudes of mind. When circumstances trigger discontent—for example, while holding a hip-opening āsana—with mindfulness practice we learn to disentangle the direct sensations from the familiar feeling of irritation or resistance to what is happening. We suspend immediately acting out from these feelings by trying to improve the posture or by coming out of it in order to avoid these feelings. When mindfulness is added to our āsana practice, we develop an increasingly spontaneous ability to pause and soften into our experience as we connect to what is arising within us, even when what we are connecting to is the feeling of tension in the body or mind.

Without a daily intention in our practice to observe ourselves with kind yet keen attention, our "ordinary" moments will continue to be driven by the habits of our conditioned responses. And that, as we may already know, is a recipe for unhappiness. If instead we educate ourselves to turn the lens inward, a kind of magic can occur. It is not the fantasy of glibly assuming that our practice will make us immune to difficulty. It is simpler and more realistic than that. It's the magic available in any ordinary moment when we attend to what is occurring in our body and mind in an uncontrived and authentic way. The result is that we untie the inner constriction, instead of seeking to eradicate the object of disdain. This enables an opportunity for liberation at any given moment. Let's look at how habits operate and how our Yoga practice can become a place to develop mindfulness.

Each moment in our lives we are faced with stimuli that our sensitive organism registers as sensations and subtle feelings that operate in a wavelike manner; pleasant and unpleasant events arise, build, and then crest, before diminishing and eventually evaporating, only to arise again, alternating as conditions shift and reconfigure. We naturally react to these pleasing and disturbing features with attraction toward that which we like, and repulsion to what we don't. Finally and quite unconsciously we move toward that which we are attracted to, and away from that which repels us.

These four beats are so swiftly passing through us each moment, we usually fail to notice they are really four distinct mind moments: stimulus, evaluation of unpleasant versus pleasant, reaction, and then action. We are often left wondering how we got here and why we are suffering without knowing there is any choice in how we relate to the recognition of unpleasant and pleasant experiences. Mindfulness is a practice that begins with the fourth beat, refraining from action. The first two, stimulus and assessment of stimulus as pleasant or unpleasant, are unavoidable and outside our control. But the second two (reaction and action) are under our conscious control, and can only be developed with training.

In mindfulness meditation, we pause the fourth beat, the action, in order to observe reactions (the third beat) to pleasant and unpleasant stimulus. Initially, this is a lot like restraining a colt. We may be bucking and rearing in discontent, but we hold our seat so that we can observe the process of reactivity a little closer. We may begin to see that distraction and discontent often arise when we are experiencing unpleasant sensations that are at the apex point, at their peak of intensity. Instead of acting out from this repulsion (however slight), and moving our attention away from what we don't want, we simply observe the feelings and sensations directly. Inevitably, we notice that what seemed solid and permanent is actually fluctuating, giving us experiential insight into the wavelike nature of change. We learn that when we can stay more attentive to both pleasant and unpleasant experiences alike, without drowning in the common hindrances of craving or aversion, we feel more alive and connected, even when what we are connecting to is difficult to endure.

The beauty of a mindfulness practice is that we can actually learn to rest in awareness even when feeling highly uncomfortable. Our attitude can become one of wonderment rather than abandonment. "Wow, look at this," might be the inner dialogue, instead of "No, I refuse to accept this." This shift in perspective allows our inner experience to become much more fluid, flexible, and adaptable. The habit of resistance to what's happening may still continue to arise, but our newfound skill to observe rather than fight or flee frees us from the prolonged damage unconscious reactivity promotes.

Mindfulness practice is taught in four domains of attention; to the body, to feelings, to mind states, to phenomenon. I have found that slower āsana practices can be a potent container in which to develop mindfulness meditation since we encounter all the same qualities of inattention or aggression when we practice holding Yoga postures as we would when meditating.

When we place ourselves in a Yoga pose, we are often so focused on the body shape we are trying to create, that we may not even notice our current attitude. We may be unaware that we are feeling frustrated by our limited range of motion in our hips or tight hamstrings, unaware that we are unintentionally inhibiting the flow of energy because of our rigid attitude. Since prāṇa (energy) flows where our soft attention goes, how we practice is as important as what we practice. The congested areas of the body interrupt our natural energy flow, but so does our rigid attitude. If we approach our tight regions with care, we can relax the struggle with our experience and really enjoy coming home to our bodies in a dignified way, regardless of our limitations.

When we practice Yoga and mindfulness of the body simultaneously, we set up a quality of genuine acceptance toward our experience. This allows insights to filter through our ordinary states of consciousness that bleed into how we live ordinary moments. On that day of infernal heat, my reaction started out as self-righteousness. I felt I had already experienced my hot flash for the hour, so I did not feel I deserved to have to go through the internal burning again. In my view, it was wrong. This contracted attitude caused me to perceive the heat as even more unendurable. The healthy habit developed from my mindfulness practice to pause and acknowledge how I was relating to my experience eventually arose and allowed me to see my responsibility for my unhappiness. I was promoting my own suffering.

Becoming aware of our habitual patterns during our practice life helps us see that living in defiance of ordinary moments like the one I have described is a choice. At the height of tension and discontent, the crest of the wave, the challenge becomes to attempt to look at and accept the feelings of rejection we are experiencing in relation to unpleasant circumstances, rather than striving to get rid of the resistance to what we don't like. As we turn openly toward our hostility without scorn or pretense, acceptance itself shifts our experience.

In mindfulness practice we are neither controlling what is happening to us, nor wallowing in resignation of our fate. We are simultaneously accepting what is here, and allowing room for the potential of change. This attitude becomes the foundation for authenticity and discriminating wisdom to develop. When something horrible is happening to us, we meet aversion in a truthful way. If it is true that I am feeling resentful, then turning toward rather than away from these feelings and allowing them to move through me without censorship is the practice of mindful awareness

When we can include rather than deny or fight with what is really true within us, the emotion becomes a little more porous. We can then inhabit the feeling consciously, discovering how every feeling feels inside our body. While we are exploring the immediate body sensations, we also relax believing the story we might be telling ourselves, whether we are justifying, blaming, or feeding self-condemnation for having these feelings. Instead of analyzing, we stay with the direct immediacy of our experience as it is unfolding in the body, giving our feelings room to breathe. Since emotions are not static, we will naturally notice how they morph into other feelings. As they shift, we continue to allow these changes without self-definition. In this way we learn to know anger or sadness directly, free of creating a permanent self or me out of them. We remain fluid within our moments, with a wider range of capacity for allowing the totality of human emotions to move through us.

As we begin our āsana practice, we acknowledge that challenges will indeed arise, and that we plan neither to cause harm to ourselves nor to abandon the scene. Temporarily (you might even say artificially), we learn to suspend the behavior that would usually result in us pushing, fighting, or running away from what is happening. Āsana practice is a perfect setting for this training since certain positions will inevitably trigger challenges. While we are experiencing various sensations, we see if we can apply the method of mindfulness directly, in our own immediate experience.

As we begin the practice, it is helpful to clearly understand the method. The first tool of mindfulness of the body is to track the in- and out- breath without interfering with its cycles. Although breath awareness can seem too dull or ordinary to elicit any insights, there are features in the breath that can teach us simple truths about life.

As we take a breath in, it feels good, particularly when it is a fresh, oxygenated breath. As we inhale, the body feels a natural relief. Then as the breath continues to come in, we usually take it for granted. After pleasure at the beginning of the in-breath, we are now feeling more indifferent. As we get to the end of the inhale, the longer we go without breathing out, the more uncomfortable it gets. It was great in the beginning, we didn't really care so much in the middle, and now we really want it to end and something else to occur. This pattern of pleasant, neutral, and unpleasant within one cycle of breath is ubiquitous in all cycles of all experience. It's a kind of arc we are exposed to in all of our waking moments. So to watch this patterning inside us breeds particular experiential insights that can translate to other encounters. Establishing the breath as our primary anchor also gives us a trustworthy base of support to return to when we either disconnect with our experience or become entangled in it.

There are outer, inner, and innermost levels of method to every practice. In mindfulness of the body, the outer or foundation level of training is to know what is happening while it is happening, to know something is changing, or to know its absence, in a noninterfering way. (The inner level of training focuses on impermanence, and the innermost is a direct recognition of emptiness.) Let's look at how this applies in our Yoga poses. The foundation level of mindfulness while in a back bend may involve paying attention to all kinds of events throughout the body and mind. On the physical level, there may be the feeling of compression (this is the word for "bones pressed closer together is not a bad thing") along the back of the spine and elongation along the front. On the emotional level we might notice trepidation and unease, while mentally we may observe we are talking to ourselves incessantly, wondering whether we should go further or come out, or we may be caught up in the memory of an event where we injured our spine.

The first method of mindfulness of the body is to disentangle the direct and immediate sensation in the body from our mental processes and reactions to the sensation. We attempt to place the sensation itself in the foreground and fully observe it, while allowing our likes and dislikes, thoughts and fantasies, to be noticed and let go of. We are not pretending we like unpleasant sensations. We are instead fully observing the nature of the sensations at hand instead of fixating on whether they are good or bad, right or wrong (unless of course we are sure it is simply risky to be in this pose).

Working with what is most difficult at the moment can allow us to stay in the process of mindfulness before any mental agitation hijacks our commitment to observe. We look into the experience more microscopically and discover the size and shape of the sensation, noticing how it feels on inhale versus exhale, and whether or not it stays the same or is shifting as we watch. This simple movement from identification with pain to observation of discomforting sensations shifts our experience completely. We might have the insight that it is easy for us to become caught in a struggle with our experience, or to become engrossed in concepts about our experience, or just to simply space out.

Maintaining an attitude of intrepid curiosity and inquiry moment to moment is an essential component to preserving mindfulness. While folding forward or bending back we can nourish this inspired attitude during our āsana time by first simply noticing pressure in the external hip rotators, thickness in the groins, or hardness in the abdomen as we bend into a hip-opening forward bend.

Secondly, we investigate how it feels specifically within the sensation itself. Instead of shifting our attention at this point, we penetrate the experience a little further. We go directly into the outer hips and notice the size and shape of the sensation. Is it stronger over on the right end or is the center more intense? Is it more oblong or rectangular? What's the texture feel like? And how is it changing moment to moment?

Lastly, we ask what's my attitude toward this experience? Once you've recognized that there's a distinction between the raw event of sensations and how you're actually relating to what's happening, you gently acknowledge the current attitude. We might feel frustration, resentment, hope, or fear. At this stage it is very important that we not censure our feelings and instead simply and nonjudgmentally, recognize what is arising within us, even when we would prefer to feel otherwise. As we accept our psychological condition with honesty and care, we can then come back to the first step and ask ourselves anew, where am I feeling this in my body? As we are investigating the various sensations within us, pose by pose, we keep coming back to the breath as our primary anchor and domain of stability.

When we give ourselves time for this noninvasive and nonabandoning quality of mindful attention during our Yoga practice each day, our relationship to ourselves becomes naturally kinder, softer, and more intimate. This primary method of mindfulness of the body develops greater ease of being under a myriad of conditions, laying a foundation of maturity in the yogic practitioner and readying us for deeper inquiry into the nature of change—the inner method of mindfulness—and eventually stimulating direct insight into the empty nature of all phenomena—the innermost path.

8

BRAHMĀ VIHĀRA, EMPTINESS, AND ETHICS

CHRISTOPHER KEY CHAPPLE

THIS CHAPTER WILL explore three points of contact between Buddhism and classical Yoga: the Brahmā Vihāra, emptiness, and ethics. All three practices lead to a goal held in common by both traditions: dharma-megha samādhi, or the "cloud of virtue" state of concentration. In Buddhist tradition, this term describes the tenth and final stage (bhūmi) of the bodhisattva path. In Yoga, this term is used to describe the state of liberation in which all afflicted action (kliṣṭa-karma) ceases.

The Brahmā Vihāra

SUKHA MAITRĪ, DUḤKHA KARUṆĀ, PUṆYA MUDITA, APUṆYA UPEKṢĀ

Be friendly with the happy, compassionate toward those
who suffer.
Celebrate the success of the virtuous, be even-minded
toward those who lack virtue.[1]

The Brahmā Vihāra system exists in both Yoga and Buddhism. In Buddhism, it describes the spontaneous actions taken by the Arhats, the five hundred individuals who attained nirvāṇa after receiving the teachings of the Buddha. The *Yoga Sūtra* inclusion of the Brahmā Vihāra indicates the influence of Buddhist meditation teachings on Patañjali, who most likely composed his text almost six hundred years after the death of the Buddha. The sūtras serve as a handbook summarizing meditation techniques current in Patañjali's time, during which Buddhist monasticism was widely known and Nalanda, the great Buddhist university, was flourishing.

In this exploration of the Brahmā Vihāra, their import will be explored using linguistic clues and word placement within the *Yoga Sūtra.* First, it can be seen that the four practices of friendliness (sometimes translated as loving-kindness), compassion, sympathetic joy (translated above as celebration of success), and equanimity (even-mindedness) do not exist as independent virtues to be applied in all instances. A context is given for each that requires discernment. When approaching people, either well known or strangers, the Buddhist or yogi is encouraged to assess their circumstance and situation. Are they in a place of happiness? Sorrow? Virtue? Viciousness? Clearly, this text values the insight required to make this assessment and encourages the practitioner to develop appropriate response behaviors. According to Richard Gombrich, the Arhats would practice this as part of the natural flow of their enlightened state. For others, it might require considerable effort.

Throughout the history of contemplative philosophy, numerous analytical systems for cultural and personality assessment have been developed, from the tuning systems and political structures described in Plato's *Republic* to the typologies of "left-brain and right-brain." The Brahmā Vihāra outlines a fourfold assessment of the human condition, placing individuals into four categories: the happy, the suffering, the virtuous, and those who lack virtue. These may be seen as either transient states or overall personality types, though no one single person could ever manifest solely one of these qualities to the exclusion of all others. Another well-known system of personality discernment, the Enneagram, suggests that by understanding nine standard personality types, one can achieve greater self-understanding as well as understanding of and hence compassion for others.[2] The latter chapters of the *Bhagavad Gītā* devote dozens of verses wherein the Avatāra Krishna instructs the warrior Arjuna about how to categorize people in terms of the three modes or guṇas: being illumined (sattva), driven by passion (rājas), or sunken into lethargy (tamas).

India abounds with lists and categories, not for their own sake, but to provide a frame for organizing one's experience of the world. All of this effort is undertaken in order for one to gain a perspective that will reduce one's investment and attachment, to move from anxiety into the more reserved stance of the observer. Hence, the Brahmā Vihāra set forth a twofold practice. First, take a step back and think about the company one keeps. Is this individual or group manifesting a place or space or mood (bhava) that merits my friendliness and hence ease (sukha)? Is this a situation wherein people are exhibiting a great need for comfort and protection and solace (duḥkha)? Is this a situation that can engender a response of jealousy or envy (puṇya)? Is this a situation that might draw one into impure acts or criminal activity (apuṇya)? By using caution and taking a second look, confidence can be gained in regard to the best path to pursue.

Another interesting aspect of the Brahmā Vihāra practice can be seen in Patañjali's choice of words. Each of the terms for these four practices carries a feminine ending: *maitrī*, *karuṇā*, *mudita*, *upekṣā*. Throughout his description of meditation practices in the first section of the *Yoga Sūtra,* Patañjali purposefully chooses words in the feminine gender.[3] In the philosophies of Sāṅkhya and Tantra, the divine feminine (prakṛti/shakti) serves two functions: experience and liberation. By highlighting the role of practice as applied in everyday life through the Brahmā Vihāra, Patañjali affirms the importance of ongoing engagement with and purification of one's involvement with the world, which expresses itself through a creativity that is deemed feminine. In later traditions specific goddesses become associated with levels of spiritual accomplishment.[4] Women in the form of bodhisattvas such as Tārā and

Kuan Yin as well as heroic human women, real and in folklore, underscore the fascination with and importance of the feminine in the broad legacy of India's spiritual traditions.

Emptiness: Śūnya and Śūnyatā

The most concise articulation of Buddhist emptiness can be found in the *Heart Sūtra,* the *Hrdaya Sūtra.* Known and beloved and memorized and chanted in Buddhist communities throughout Asia, it has been rendered by Philip Kapleau as follows:

> The Bodhisattva of Compassion, from the depths of Prajñā Wisdom, saw the emptiness of all five skandhas, and sundered the bonds of suffering. Form here is only emptiness, emptiness only form. Form is no other than emptiness, emptiness no other than form. Feeling, thought and choice, consciousness itself, are the same as this.
>
> Dharmas here are empty, all are the primal void. None are born or die, nor are they stained or pure, nor do they wax or wane. So in emptiness no form, no feeling, thought, or choice, nor is there consciousness. No eye, ear, nose, tongue, body, mind; no color, sound, smell, taste, touch, or what the mind takes hold of, nor even act of sensing. No ignorance or end of it, nor all that comes of ignorance; no withering, no death, no end of them. Nor is there pain or cause of pain or cease in pain or noble path to lead from pain, not even wisdom to attain, attainment too is emptiness.[5]

This hymn encapsulates the insights of both Abhidharma and Mādhyamika philosophy, outlining the basic teachings of the Buddha and the philosopher Nagarjuna. The Buddha proclaimed that suffering results from desire. Desire is enacted through the senses and the body. The senses and the body are not linked to an enduring soul but to an aggregate of ever-changing combinations of form, feeling, thought, choice (karmic residue), and momentary flashes of consciousness. By disengaging identification with any particular fixed moment, including moments of self-claimed spiritual attainment, a freedom flows forth characterized as empty (śūnya) or free from clinging.

Patañjali also takes up this term. In several passages he applauds emptiness (śūnya) as the supreme accomplishment of Yoga. In the first section of the book he proclaims that when one is able to purify the memory of karmic influence, the core purpose of an object shines forth. All objects exist for the sake of bringing one to a state of purified consciousness. When this takes place, it is as if the prior form, the one to which one had developed attachment and clinging, becomes emptied. Patañjali states:

> *Nirvitarka* (a state of *samādhi* wherein one becomes freed from reliance on external objects for concentration) is when memory is purified, as if emptied of own-form, and the purpose alone shines forth.[6]

This moment of absorptive awareness renders the particular cluster of factors that give rise to name and form inoperable; Patañjali describes this moment as having unity among grasper, grasping, and grasped.

This experience of emptiness and its link to the goal and purpose of Yoga is restated in Patañjali's description of samādhi:

> When the purpose alone shines forth,
> as if empty of own form,
> that indeed is *samādhi*.[7]

By overcoming the tendency to hold on to the past or overly anticipate the future due to karmic impressions, then one becomes ripe for release.

Continuing this theme, the very final passage of the *Yoga Sūtra* describes this experience in light of guṇa theory (mentioned earlier), the release into blessed aloneness (kaivalyam), and the assertion of the presence of higher consciousness (citi-śakti), a concept that again reinforces the importance of the feminine in Yoga. The process of emptying remains central to this culminating moment:

> The return to the origins of the *guṇas* (signifying that the creative dance of *prakṛti* has ceased), emptied of their purpose for *puruṣa* (the pure consciousness), is *kaivalyam*, the steadfastness in own-form, and the power of higher awareness.[8]

Each of these three sūtra*s* include the Buddhist term *śūnya,* the cornerstone of Mahāyāna philosophy. As with Buddhism, Patañjali asserts that one must clean out all occasions for attachment through self-understanding and practice. Unlike the Buddhism of the *Heart Sūtra,* Patañjali suggests that this delivers one to a higher state of awareness, though he is also careful to warn that this "higher mind" cannot be seen:

> In trying to see another, higher mind
> there is an overstretching of the intellect
> from the intellect and a confusion of memory.[9]

Like the author of the *Heart Sūtra,* Patañjali knows that one cannot state positively one's own attainment of wisdom.

Ethics

Yoga, Buddhism, and Jainism all share a common code, with slight variations. Its earliest written mention can be found in the *Ācāranga Sūtra* (ca. 350 B.C.E.), where Mahāvīra, regarded by the Jainas to be their twenty-fourth and most recent great teacher, proclaimed five principles to be followed: nonviolence, truthfulness, not stealing, sexual restraint, and nonpossession. Patañjali follows these exactly without variation. The Buddhist teachers place not stealing before truthfulness, and replace nonpossession with abstention from all intoxicants.

In all three traditions, the intent of ethical practice remains constant. All three systems seek release from suffering caused by karmic impulses. According to Patañjali, the benefits are immense. From overcoming violence, all animosity ceases in one's presence. From telling the truth, reliability results. From overcoming covetousness, all things become like jewels. From sexual restraint, great vigor arises. And when one owns little, the origins of all things become clear.[10]

This first list of precepts advises one to abstain from activities that generate negative karma. The second, complementary pathway within Yoga, known as the observances (niyāma), prescribes positive behaviors, by which one builds a reserve of virtue. Buddhism develops a somewhat parallel practice in its advocacy of the six perfections (pāramitā). Patañjali describes purity, contentment, austerity, study, and dedication to Īśvara (the special being never touched by karma) as key to the cultivation of purified karmas. Buddhism lists six perfections: giving, proper behavior, patience, strength, wisdom, and meditation. By aligning the Sanskrit terms for each, we can see some similarities in the strategies employed to overcome negative karma.

The Buddhist practice of giving or generosity (dāna) has no direct parallel in the Yoga lists, though in the process of practicing the renunciation of possessions (aparigraha) one might give away various items. The first of Patañjali's observances, śauca, or purified action, aligns well with the Buddhist practice of śīla, or proper behavior. By being upright in all activity, one cultivates positive actions or karmas. The second of the niyāmas, contentment (santoṣa), finds similarity to the third Buddhist perfection, patience (kṣānti). The third, austerity (tapas), often requires periods of fasting and silence. These generate heat within the body that serves the physical function of burning off the subtle residues of karma. In Buddhism, the perfection of strength (vīrya) serves a similar function. The study of texts that refer to the highest self (svādhyāyā) correlates to the adoption of the wisdom view (prajñā), the fifth of the Buddhist perfections. For Patañjali, the wisdom (prajñā) described in the first section of the *Yoga Sūtra* brings one to an elevated state of moving within the great order and beauty of life: ṛtambharā tatra prajñā, which may be translated as "There, the wisdom bears the cosmic rhythm (*ṛta*)."[11]

The fifth of Patañjali's observances, dedication to Īśvara, requires an emptying of oneself through extended contemplation of an exalted ideal who has never fallen under the sway of karma: "Perfection in samādhi arises from dedication to Īśvara" (*YS* II.45). For the Buddhists, this Īśvara would be figure of the Buddha himself, who successfully examined and understood and went beyond all his past and present karmas. To meditate within Buddhism, the sixth and final perfection, draws one into an emulation of the Buddha himself, the exemplary meditator. Patañjali suggests that one can choose any deity (iṣṭa devatā) just as he also suggests that one can take on any object for one's meditation practice ("Or from meditation as desired," yathā abhimata-dhyānād-vā[12]).

In both Buddhism and in Patañjali's classical Yoga, these positive cultivations of auspicious karma help set one free.

Practice

Each of these three examples of the Brahmā Vihāra, the philosophy of emptiness and cultivation of a life informed and guided by ethical decision making, carries practical applications. Drawing from my own experience as a student and teacher of Yoga and meditation, some stories and examples will be given for each that might resonate with the reader.

In regard to the practice of the Brahmā Vihāra, I will share a story that helped me understand the importance of discernment when choosing to place oneself in the company of others. The first story pertains to the "sizing up of others" aspect of this practice, by way of my first extended encounter with a senior monk of the Theravāda Buddhist tradition. In the early 1980s, I invited Venerable Guṇaratana to speak on the campus of Stony Brook University. Bhante came from a very poor Sri Lankan family and had risen to become one of the great scholars and meditation teachers of the Theravāda tradition. In 1968 he founded the Washington, D.C., Buddhist Vihāra and served as spiritual advisor to countless immigrants and Americans who came to embrace Buddhist meditation. Following his concise and inspirational lecture on the nature of Buddhist philosophy and the purpose of meditation, the room was open for questions. One student asked an incredibly rude, challenging question that confronted and ridiculed the very premises of Buddhism. With aplomb and without missing a beat, Venerable Guṇaratana acknowledged that the ideas of Buddhism might not fit with the student's worldview, quietly restated the goal of Buddhism, and moved on to the next question. Later, back at the office, I apologized (probably overlyprofusely) for the student's bad manners; as host, I felt mortified that such an unfortunate interchange had taken place. Bhante quickly put me at ease, and instructed me about the nature of questions. He explained that one of the things he learned from the Abhidharma philosophical tradition was that the questioner is always more important than the question. One type of questioner merely asks the question to demonstrate his or her own knowledge, relevant or not, to the topic at hand. The second type of questioner has no particular point of view, but wants only to confront and belittle. The third type of questioner, the most rare of all, comes from a genuine place of seeking knowledge. This assessment helped me immensely. Not only did Bhante's words put me at ease in regard to my hospitality, they have also proven useful in the university classroom and in my various roles as a meditation teacher.

For twelve years my wife and I were core members of Yoga Anand Ashram and disciples of Gurani Añjali, an Indian meditation teacher from Calcutta. For thousands of hours we sat with her, learning about ourselves, learning about the world, and meeting a variety of challenges, large and small.[13] Having started Yoga training at a young age during my first year of university, I was, on reflection, a bit vulnerable and, like many people in my stage of life, trying to find my way. A simple piece of advice stayed with me over these many years: choose friends and companions who will bring you strength and complement your weaknesses; spend your time with those who will lift you up, not bring you down. These words attuned me to paying attention to the mood and intentions of others, to discern personalities in such a way that would help me avoid trouble. As with the Brahmā Vihāra, where advice is given about how to manage people in four different contexts, so this attentiveness to personality types has girded me with an ability to choose the company of like-minded people, while of course, as a teacher and professor, not ignoring the needs of others. Friendliness toward the good and rejoicing in the accomplishments of others has helped cultivate the strength needed when attempting to compassionately help those who suffer and to remain in equanimity when disappointed or let down by people who behave badly.

Emptiness (śūnyatā) puzzled me in the early days of practice and study. While an undergraduate, I had the good fortune to study with a direct original disciple of Geshe Wangyal, the Mongolian teacher of Tibetan Buddhism who trained the first generation of Buddhist scholar-practitioners, including Robert Thurman, Jeffrey Hopkins, Anne Klein, and others. My teacher, Christopher Starr George, having dropped out of Harvard in the early 1960s, traveled with his friend, Bob Thurman, to central New Jersey to learn Tibetan language and philosophy from Geshe Wangyal, part of a group of refugees given haven by the Tolstoy Foundation. George completed his doctorate at the University of Pennsylvania by translating portions of the *Caṇḍamahāroṣaṇa Tantra* under the tutelage of a lama in Nepal, and started teaching Tibetan and Sanskrit at Stony Brook University through the Institute for Advanced Studies of World Religions. We read many chapters of the *Bodhicaryavatāra* of Śāntideva and various passages of Nagarjuna, simultaneously in Sanskrit and Tibetan. My polyglot fellow student Ken Meyer followed along by reading the Chinese as well. From this exposure, we delved into the standard Buddhist critiques of self and explored the philosophical function of the Buddha's assertion of no-self. This inquiry did remain in the realm of academic speculation, but carried over into reflections on daily life.

Many years ago, as newlyweds, my wife and I were grappling with the everyday problems of simply getting along and went to Añjali for counseling. She advised us to simply surrender to the other, to be of service to each other, in a sense to use the ability to become empty vessels. In those early months, we realized that despite our intimacy, we remain separate individuals, supporting each other yet with distinct paths. Years later, my friend and student Donovan Duket traveled from Los Angeles to take her darśhan at the ashram. In response to her invitation to ask her a question, he sheepishly told about moving back in with his mother after graduating from college, and having a very hard time adjusting to her little requests. Añjali laughed and said, "She is your mother! If she asks you to take out the garbage, just take out the garbage!" By surrendering resistance, we move into a place of emptying, a place of release from ego, a giving up to the other that provides liberation from the binding nature of self. Emptiness, seemingly lofty and abstract in the literature of Buddhism and Yoga, has a direct application and utility in daily life.

A breakthrough in understanding emptiness in relation to puruṣa came in the form of an insight that Buddhism and Yoga, although using different terminology, point to a similar state of transcendence. All states of identification (asmitā) and pride (abhimāna) stem from attachment due to the afflictions (kleśa) of karma. For me, the experience of puruṣa has come from the wearing away of tendencies to cling to fixed notions of how things should be, for both myself and others. By relinquishing comparison and judgment, a feeling of ease with others has emerged. This constitutes an ongoing practice that, in Buddhist terms, reveals the underlying emptiness of constructed phenomena. As parents, we have guided a son and daughter to adulthood while recognizing their autonomy in their life choices. My thinking mind can be riven with my own hopes and expectations for them, leading to anxiety. Only when I relinquish these projections and imaginings can I fully enjoy and celebrate their accomplishments and gifts.

Ethics form the core of meditation practice. The precepts and observances listed earlier anchor classical Yoga as taught in the tradition in which I was trained. My first exposure to this form of Yoga came through asking about a word: *ahiṁsā*. A classmate, Carole Zeiler, had spent her senior year of high school taking Yoga classes with Añjali, just prior to the dedication of the ashram in 1972. As we became friends,

I learned from Carole about the yamas and niyāmas, about how to aspire to be nonviolent in thought, word, and deed; to be honest; to not steal time or status from others; to be careful about acquiring possessions; to be clean; to be austere; to be studious; in short, how to cultivate a life grounded in spiritual principles.[14] By forging patterns of positive behaviors, the lethargy and attachments of earlier youthful indiscretions slowly lessened their grip, allowing for a lighter sense of self to emerge. These ten touchstones, which I still assign weekly to my own Yoga students in Santa Monica, prepare one to confront the challenges of both one's own karmic density and the attachments of others.

Conclusion: Dharma Megha Samādhi

The *Dasabhūmika Sūtra* of Mahāyāna Buddhism (ca. 300 C.E.) states that at the tenth and final stage of the path, one enters dharma megha samādhi. In this state, one "acquires a glorious body . . . emits rays which destroy the pain and misery of all living beings . . . cultivates the perfection of knowledge (jñāna) without neglecting others."[15] Vijnāna Bhikṣu, a sixteenth-century commentator on Yoga, states that the one who is "established in *dharma megha samādhi* is called a liberated soul (*jīvan mukta*)."[16] From this place, one no longer creates karma that binds oneself or other people. Rather than taking, one is able to give freely. By knowing the contexts of our interactions, by surrendering attachments to ideas of self-importance and resistance to others, and by using precepts and positive behaviors as the guideposts for behavior, Yoga and Buddhism suggest pathways for self-purification, allowing one to act in accord with dharma and be of service to others.

9

BUDDHA AND THE YOGI

Paradigms of Restraint and Renunciation

MU SOENG

THE WORDS *YOGA* and *mindfulness* (here understood as a derivative of Buddhist thought and practice) have not only entered the lexicon of popular culture in America in recent years but seem also to have accommodated themselves to a familiar pattern of commodification in which a trend or an idea becomes validated only by its status as an item of conspicuous consumption. There's a certain strangeness to this pattern in which Yoga or mindfulness is seen as a matter of branding, and essentially not different from, say, branding and selling coffee or dish soap on cable TV—different props in pursuit of a self-defined level of comfort and ease. But to those who have done some in-depth study and practice of Yoga and mindfulness, something seems to be missing; something fundamental to the raison d'être of both traditions. In their long history in Asia, both traditions have been seen as road maps for a way of living—a disciplined daily life molded and modified according to a shared core principle of letting go; not clinging; not hankering after the things of the world.

While the application of Yoga as a promoter of good health and of Buddhist mindful meditation as a stress reducer are uncontroversial and welcome, there's also a sense that there's more to them than their current status as mere consumer items. For one thing, in the classical tradition of Yoga in India, Hatha Yoga (physical postures, or āsanas), taught today in a "Yoga studio" in almost every neighborhood in America, is only a small part of the larger culture of Yoga. Physical fitness and toning the body are only a beginning step; the broader framework is to begin to see the things of the world not as items of consumption but as a place of ultimate unsatisfactoriness.

Similarly, Buddhist mindfulness practice encompasses much more than the simple idea of stress reduction and includes a much larger vision of the individual and society. Thus, there's a sense that much can be learned from how the two traditions have served as a "civilizational" guidepost in the long history of Asia. When we sort through various layers of doctrines and practices in both traditions, we find that what binds them both is a shared vision of individuals and society grounded in restraint and renunciation, in simplicity, in doing away with the clutter of possessions, and so on. This vision is also shared by the Taoists in China.

And this is where the real problem of assimilating these two traditions into the mainstream culture of America begins. There's a fundamental clash of worldviews in these two traditions with those of the Judeo-Christian worldview. The success so far, admittedly limited and largely as consumer items, of these two traditions has come mainly through their embrace by secularists, who are not so beholden to the Judeo-Christian worldviews. The pliability of the Buddhist and yogic worldviews allows them not only to be susceptible to aggressive marketing strategies but also nonthreatening to the Judeo-Christian worldview.

If the purpose of philosophy or religion is to shape the lives of individuals so that they may live together more harmoniously and creatively as a society, then the function of restraint and renunciation, championed by both traditions, is "civilizational" in the sense of shaping the lives of the individuals and society through simplicity and nonattachment. The premise of restraint and renunciation calls upon individuals to let go of their inherited religious dogmas and ideologies, to let go of the impulse to exploit and harm others, to let go of the desire to maximize one's own pleasure at the expense of others, and to focus instead on the ethical cohesion of daily living. In this argument, an ethically cohesive individual is a healthy individual who becomes both the cause and the effect of a healthy society.

The Buddhist and Yoga traditions both warn repeatedly against the dangers of greed, hatred, and delusion, and promote a culture of restraint and renunciation as a counterbalance to these dangers. But if promoters of Buddhism or Yoga in the contemporary "marketplace" use the familiar but unexamined drives of greed to promote their own "product" when the culture is already permeated in greed, the end result will likely be that both of these traditions become passing fads in the great streaming of American consumerism. In the unexamined patterns of defining themselves as "service providers," the spiritual entrepreneurs in both traditions may end up marginalizing the larger role that these two traditions can possibly play in the shaping of the culture. Right now it seems we need all the counterweight we can gather to meet the challenge of unbridled greed promoted by American consumerism.

In the long history of Indian religious and philosophical thought—in which Buddhism and Yoga are joined at the hip—there is a shared understanding that saṃsāra, the conditioned human existence, is a place of sorrow and despair. While the two traditions differ in their methodologies of transcending saṃsāra, there's also a shared understanding that the greatest human achievement is to work on one's own negative patterns and dispositions so that one achieves the "goal" of not being reborn into saṃsāra. While this conventional goal flirts with metaphysical speculations, there's a self-evident existential dimension to an individual's wholehearted commitment to work on healing the negative aspects of his or her conditioning. And this existential dimension is what resonates most for a thoughtful, reflective contemporary person while engaged with these two ancient traditions.

The Sanskrit word *saṃsāra* literally means "journeying" or "wandering on," as in wandering endlessly in the rounds of birth, death, rebirth. Thus, in a strict sense, saṃsāra is not a place but a process: the processes of craving and clinging; of greed, hatred, and delusion.

In both Buddhist and Yoga traditions, saṃsāra is synonymous with conditioned existence, which in turn is experienced as painful, unsatisfactory, and not capable of providing a taste of true and lasting happiness. The patterns of greed, hatred, and delusion are the building blocks of saṃsāra in that they keep one hooked into craving for "more." This distrust is allied with another shared worldview: that the end of craving and clinging will come about through letting go, through cultivating restraint and renunciation in one's own life as well as in the life of the collective entity.

It remains undisputed that when the Buddha left home at the age of twenty-nine to enter the forest, he stepped into a culture and community of wandering ascetics (Pali: samana; Skt: śramaṇa). By all accounts, it was a vibrant and vital culture at the time; and historians are intrigued by the fact that even at such an early period in human history it was such a distinct part of Indian culture.[1]

Today we recognize this culture of wandering ascetics as part of a "Yoga" tradition that goes back even further into the reaches of Indian prehistory. What remains astonishing, too, is the fact that this ancient sensibility has remained an integral part of Indian religious and cultural tradition down to the present day. India remains perhaps the only society in the world where a naked sannyāsin (ascetic) can walk nonchalantly through the streets of a metropolis and not only not be harmed or jeered at but be accorded a certain degree of acceptance and respect.[2] Thus, a nuance of "Yoga," within both the Buddhist tradition and the larger Indian religious tradition, goes beyond a mere counting of schools or lineages or religious slogans or philosophical doctrines. "Yoga," as an indicator of a society's spiritual health, remained a sort of underground stream in most Asian societies until recent times, and it can properly be defined as a promoter of a culture of restraint and renunciation.

The links of the śramaṇa culture of the Buddha's time to an even more ancient tradition of Yoga remain less than clear but are definitive. We know today of the discovery of a seal from the ruins of the pre-Aryan civilization of Mohenjodaro (ca. 2500 B.C.E.) that shows a person sitting in a cross-legged position of yogic meditation. Everything else about the origins of Yoga is a matter of speculation and conjecture; so, too, is our understanding of Indian religious culture before the time of the Buddha. The myths and legends of India (contained largely in its Purāṇa literature), as well as the organization of the society contained in the *Vedas,* suggest the possibility of two competing "value systems" at a very early state: one that adopted Śiva, the "god of asceticism," as its model, and another that adopted Viṣṇu, the "householder's god," as its iconic figure. These two competing ideas, in their various permutations and combinations, have continued to inform Indian religious identities down to this day.

Given what we know about the śramaṇa culture at the time of the Buddha, it can be said that it was a culture of extreme asceticism. This association of Yoga with extreme asceticism has remained more or less constant down to this day. In this version, Yoga is a free-form pursuit of gaining magical powers. The worldview of pre-Buddhist India imagined a universe populated by various spirits—deities, nature spirits, and so on—who were "sentient" enough to be corralled by the "heat" generated through tapas or tapasya (austerity or mortification). Whoever could do these extreme austerities would have control over enormous powers and would be the king of the world. In this interpretation, the practice of extreme asceticism was a struggle for worldly power through the power of magic. Any sundry reading of the Purāṇas bears out this interpretation. In these myths, legendary ascetics such as Vaśiṣṭa, Viśvāmitra, Paraśurāma, and others were not really nice and kind people; they all wanted their commands to be obeyed by kings and commoners alike, no matter what. If these commands were not obeyed, their wrath would know no bounds.

It is worth noting that asceticism was a common feature of all ancient societies. Early Christianity was clearly influenced by even earlier forms of Egyptian and Syrian asceticism. As Joseph P. Amar, a contemporary scholar of early Christian asceticism has written,

> The heroes of this new model of ascetic life were Elijah and John the Baptist, who emptied themselves of the world to live solitary lives of mortification in the desert. Although the homily's emphasis on escape from the world and its unreserved praise of ascetic excess have more in common with the Evagrian-inspired asceticism of Egypt than with the original spirit of native Syrian asceticism, this new and rigorous model of Christian perfection would irrevocably influence and alter the earlier, more moderate impulse.[3]

A new turning in the pre-Buddhist Vedic thought came through the body of literature known as the *Upaniṣads,* which suggested a new interpretation of tapas, or the heat generated by ascetic practices. These new thinkers thought it more proper to think that this heat will burn away the ego structures and prepare the ascetic, through surrender and concentration, for merging with the universal consciousness (Brahmān) and thus gain liberation (mokṣa). This interpretation comes much closer to the Middle Way of the Buddha, and in the practical application of this interpretation the Upaniṣadic seers are willing to seek ultimate reality through wisdom and intellect rather than ascetic mortification.

Two other well-known ascetic contemporaries of the Buddha, Mahāvīra and Makkaligośāla, were renowned for their powers of asceticism. In fact, the Buddha himself became known as a champion ascetic during the six years after he left home to enter the forest. Various accounts tell us that his body became so emaciated that he could touch his backbone through his rib cage; there was no flesh left; the body had truly become a "bag of bones." These same accounts tell us that at some point he realized that all this mortification of the flesh had not brought him the inner peace he sought.

Thus, a turning point in the history of Yoga in India was reached when the Buddha realized that extreme asceticism was not necessarily going to bring him the sense of ease and well-being he was seeking. His innovation of a "middle way" between the extreme asceticism of Yoga and the indulgence of the householder within the śramaṇa culture of the day is a new departure in Indian religious history.

This Middle Way may be defined as a culture of restraint and renunciation in a balanced manner through nonclinging and nonattachment. This new culture of the middle way was a rejection of extreme asceticism but still an embrace of Yoga's sensibility of nonindulgence. Equally importantly, the Middle Way of the Buddha was a rejection of the pursuit of magical powers as a paradigm of religious life. In its place, the Buddha emphasized a pursuit of inner peace, of tranquillity, of serenity. The tools for this new pursuit were a life of nonclinging, of letting go, of restraint and renunciation, without the heavy baggage of earlier mortification practices. The life of the community that the Buddha formed around himself is an eloquent example of its acknowledged association with a new interpretation of Yoga.

The Buddha introduced a new type of meditation in the religious culture of his time, and this new meditation replaced, at least for his community of followers, the widespread practices of extreme asceticism as the methodology of liberation. This is the Middle Way of the Buddha, in which meditation, wisdom, and ethical behavior support one another in a triangular mutuality. Significant differences of doctrinal understanding, no doubt, remained between followers of Buddha's path of liberation and those on the yogic path, but they found a common cause in a culture of restraint and renunciation despite the Buddha's rejection of extreme asceticism.

Perhaps a useful way of understanding the new Middle Way of the Buddha is to see it as a "discipline" in contrast to austerities. A "discipline" is guided by a "curriculum," a graduated and interrelated set of instructions that also provide a certain measure of "progress" along the way. Over the centuries and generations in India, Yoga has also come to be seen as a "discipline" (through the eight-limbed Aṣṭāṅga Yoga) for the majority of its practitioners, except for the few diehards given to extreme austerities.

In my reading of Buddhist history, in promoting a culture of restraint and renunciation the Buddha remained within the broader confines of Yoga culture while at the same time departing from it in significant ways. As mentioned above, this departure is clearly a rejection of the pursuit of magical powers as a way of gaining worldly and religious status. It may have been the case that the geographical area where the Buddha grew up was relatively unaffected by the older Brahamānical culture of the Indo-Gangetic plains—with its yogis pursuing magical powers and its society encased in a caste system—and that he had the perspective of an outsider to the śramaṇa culture even as he was deeply immersed in it for those six years after leaving home.

But the rejection of the earlier goals of extreme asceticism did not mean that the Buddha did not see a lot of value in leaving a householder's life and adopting the ways of a wandering ascetic. In this valorization, the Buddha seemed to concur with the broader Indian idea that the world of craving and clinging—saṃsāra—was ultimately unsatisfactory and was bound to produce pain and anguish. In this way of looking at things, pursuit of, or indulgence in, food, sex, sleep, fame, and wealth diverts attention away from the higher goal of liberation. Birth in saṃsāra is unfortunate, in this view; the goal of liberation is to end the process of death and rebirth.

The mainstream culture of Buddha's time, dominated by the Brahmin priesthood, rested on the notion that the gods took an active part in the affairs of humans and that they needed to be propitiated. Such propitiation and/or protection from the wrath of the gods came through rituals and sacrifices performed by the priesthood according to ancient codes. This mainstream culture was still very fluid at the time of Buddha's birth, and a new urban culture was just barely emerging at the time. In contrast to this culture, the dropout culture of the ascetics, the precursors of what we now consider to be "Yoga," believed that only extreme asceticism will bring one to liberation.

The Buddha's corrective in this fluid environment came through the ten ascetic "dhutanga" practices he suggested to his followers. These practices are an alternative to extreme asceticism, and are a clear example that the Buddha never doubted the basic yogic principles of restraint and renunciation as the path to a life of concentration and discipline that would "shake off" the passions that so cloud the human mind. These ten practices are as follows:

1. Wearing only patched robes, that is, a robe made from discarded patches rather than new cloth
2. Not owning more than one robe with three pieces, that is, three layers of wraps
3. Eating only begged food
4. Eating only one meal a day
5. Not hoarding any food, that is, no second helping at any time of the day
6. Living in a secluded, solitary place
7. Living in a charnel ground
8. Living under a tree
9. Living in the open
10. Sleeping while sitting up, that is, never lying down to sleep[4]

By contrast, the extreme ascetic practices of Yoga would have included (if current Yoga practices in India are any indication) staring at the sun without blinking for hours at a time, or standing on one leg for months and years, or lying down on a bed of sharp nails. In the new Middle Way of the Buddha, these dhutanga practices were to be incorporated into the life of a wandering Buddhist renunciate along with the practice of the Eightfold Path, whereas a householder could focus largely on practicing the Eightfold Path while incorporating some dhutanga practices, such as eating one meal a day, in his or her daily life whenever possible. It was clearly understood in the culture of the Middle Way that the life of the wandering ascetic was most conducive to letting go of craving and clinging, for training in concentrative meditation practices, and so on.

It must be said that even though these dhutanga practices seem extreme to us moderns, especially in the West, among the hard-core śramans of the Buddha's time they may have seemed "soft." It would take a much bigger tome to parse out all the variances of their differences, but it all seems to come down to the ascetic's pursuit of magical powers that justified (to him) all the extreme austerities. For the Buddha and Buddhist monks in later generations, at least in India, the call for leaving home to enter the forest was a conscious devaluation of saṃsāra, the world of craving and clinging. The Buddhist tradition shares this common worldview with the Yoga tradition as well as an inability to understand that this devaluation may be the greatest stumbling block to a genuine understanding of what these two traditions were aspiring for.

For both traditions, a devaluation of saṃsāra is a positive hermeneutic simply because it locates itself in a directly verifiable existential system of action and consequence. If the goal of Buddhist meditation was to experience the "peace that passeth understanding," it could be done only through going inward, through disciplining breath and refining perception and cognition, rather than engagement with external things. It is also important to remember that this devaluation was not based on any nihilistic undertone but was rather an experience-based sensibility. One's actions derive from one's worldview, and if one's worldview is based on the notion that the world of craving and clinging is not satisfactory in the long run, there would be no reason to remain bound to that world. Thus, leaving home to enter the forest was not only a symbolic gesture but also a concrete choice that took one further and further away from the known world of craving and clinging.

Consider also the fact that the Buddha's definitive manual on how to do meditation practice, the *Satipaṭṭhānā Sutta* (Discourse on the Foundations of Mindfulness) contains specific practices on the foulness of the body as well as charnel-ground meditations. Their aim always was to facilitate the letting go of craving and clinging. But it also remains an interesting aspect of Buddhist history that extreme asceticism never really disappeared from the culture of the Middle Way. The Buddha may not have endorsed such practices, but in the later variations of Buddhism, such as Vajrayāna Buddhism of Tibet or Shingon Buddhism of Japan, we find a reappearance of these practices of extreme mortification. When we hear of the extremes of Milarepa's practices in Tibet or the Shingon monks standing under icy waterfalls for long periods of time, we are reminded of the vestigial residues of a very ancient impulse in the human mind regarding control, mastery, magic, domination, and so forth.

The lived reality of Buddhist thought and practice in Asia has been a series of practices, some for the monks (dhutanga practices), some for laypeople (the Eightfold Path), but both demographics nestled in a "community" of mutual support. Both the monks and laypeople were expected to embrace the culture of restraint and renunciation to the extent possible, the least of which was a life of physical and psychological simplicity. This community not only saw itself nestled within the broad sensibility of "Yoga" but also saw many overlaps between their own community and that of the Yoga practitioners.

As a correlate to the dhutanga practices of the wandering Buddhist monk, the householders who affiliated themselves with the teachings of the Buddha also embraced a life of simplicity as a derivative of the new culture of restraint and renunciation. Though these householders may still have lived surrounded by family and obligations, their choices in food, clothing, shelter, and other possessions became simpler and more austere, not given to conspicuous consumption or ostentatious display, the staple of the status-seeking householder's life. In cases where kings became converted to Buddha's teachings—such as King Ashoka in ancient India or some Burmese kings in modern times—the entire royal household reshaped itself to a simple habitat. It can be conjectured that the royal court, too, was impacted by this new way of doing things.

It is also interesting to see how the Middle Way of restraint and renunciation, developed by the Buddha, played itself out against the support systems required by the practitioners of extreme mortification. In the case of the latter, a small group of "devotees" would normally gather around the yogi and provide whatever support was needed for the yogi to continue his practice of austerity. The yogi's practice could go on for years and he would stay in one place, while the supporting cast would shift around him. In contemporary vernacular, these stationary places are called akhada, or a gathering of followers.

By contrast, the Buddhist monk was encouraged to travel through the towns, villages, and forests of ancient India for nine months of the year, never staying in one place for more than three days at a time, and staying with a group of fellow monks to practice śīla (behavioral impeccability) and samādhi (meditative discipline) during the three months of the monsoon rains. It was taken for granted by the villagers and the townspeople that these monks were practitioners of restraint and renunciation even as they carried the message of the Noble Eightfold Path of the Buddha, and hence were worthy of support through food, shelter, and medicine. But they moved on. Thus the Buddhist monk, by definition, was "faceless," not an individual personality but a model representative of a new culture of restraint and renunciation. The yogi, by contrast, was a powerhouse of an individual personality. While both have a certain stated goal—liberation or mokṣa for the ascetic; liberation or nibbāna (Skt: nirvāṇa) for the Buddhist monk—the hermeneutics of liberation might mean radically different things to each group. For the Yoga practitioner, the merging of the individual soul (Ātman) with the universal soul (Brahmān) was a positively stated goal, while for the Buddhist practitioner, the ending of the rebirth process—in whatever form or shape—was a negatively stated goal.

That the Buddha was fully committed to a culture of restraint and renunciation is testified to by the momentous decision he made to stay in the forest after his awakening experience. The importance of this decision cannot be overstated. On every count, he could have gone back to his comfortable home and family, set himself up as a "guru," and lived a life of physical ease and comfort. Yet he chose to live the life of a wandering yogi, dressed in rags and walking barefoot, negotiating the hazards and uncertainties of a forest life. Why did he choose this life?

If we accept the notion that the Buddha was a formidable intellect and innovative thinker, we should be willing to concede that it was a fully thought-out decision that resonated for him in his own personal experience. Before a community could be formed, and even before the Buddha could command the allegiance of his former colleagues, he had to convince himself beyond a shadow of doubt that a life of restraint and renunciation alone could be a container for genuine happiness, for a deeper sense of well-being, and for an authentic sense of ease.

For us moderns this is the hardest part to reconcile in the Middle Way of the Buddha: we are convinced that we can have our cake and eat it too; we can have all our toys and our comforts and yet we can be free from the workings of craving and clinging, so long as we are "mindful." In theory, it is possible, but it remains a tricky issue, and we must not underestimate the power of deceiving ourselves through our own self-rationalizations. Both the Buddhist and the Yoga tradition remain consistent in their insistence that leaving the householder's life and all its complexities is an optimal way to leave behind craving and clinging.

Even when, in the centuries after the death of the Buddha, there emerged a cadre of scholar-monks specializing in the Abhidhamma (Skt: Abhidharma) categories of analysis, they did not abandon the principle of restraint and renunciation. They seem to have lived frugally and austerely in line with the principles of the Middle Way of the Buddha except that permanent dwellings (vihāra) had become a nominative part of Buddhist communities and these scholar-monks could pursue their intellectual pursuits without the traditional wandering mores of the "preacher" monks. These monks, high-powered intellectuals all, delighted in creating and expanding the commentarial tradition and, in the process, collaborated and collided with post-Upaniṣadic thinkers in pushing the doctrinal boundaries a bit further in each generation. In that sense they were precursors of the scholar-monks of medieval Europe as also of the great Śaṅkara (788–82), the founder of Advaita Vedānta within the Hindu tradition.

Śaṅkara, considered by his followers to be an ascetic of the highest order, is also seen as a renewer of Hindu philosophical thought after nearly a thousand years of domination by Buddhist philosophers. He has also been called a closet Buddhist by his detractors. Regardless, centuries before Śaṅkara, an intimate collaboration had been initiated between Buddhists and the remnants of the yogic as well the śramaṇa cultures of ancient India. This collaboration is known today as Tantra, and its first recognizable shape, on the Buddhist side of things, seems to have emerged in late third or early fourth century C.E. It seems reasonable to conjecture that in the centuries since the time of the Buddha, "yogic" practices, meaning extreme austerities or quasi-austere practices, were very much alive within both the Buddhist and the non-Buddhist communities. It is also quite possible that these practices were numerically more widespread than were the much smaller communities of Abhidhamma scholar-monks. Certainly, the rise of Mahāyāna in late ancient and early medieval India, as a religion of faith and devotion, bears the imprint of these practices.

The "school" where the collaboration between Indian Mahāyāna Buddhism and Hindu Tantra practices first blossomed is called the Yogācāra, meaning the "application" (cāra) of Yoga. Nothing could be more evidentiary than the name of the school itself. Yogācāra is the last great unfolding of Indian Mahāyāna Buddhism, building upon the initial Prajñapāramitā schools (those who believed the Prajña-pāramitā group of sūtras as the word of the Buddha and worshiped the texts) and the Mādhyamika schools (based on the dialectical method founded by the great Nagarjuna in the second century C.E.).

Looking back at the history of early medieval Indian Buddhism, it can be seen that the Yogācāra school sought to restore the primacy of rigorous practices of meditation that was a nominative feature of the life of early Buddhist communities but that seems to have been lost or diluted in the development of the cadre of scholar-monks of the Abhidhamma or the devotional practices of the Prajña-pāramitā or the rigorous dialectic of the Mādhyamika. The Tantra arose out of and within the residual Yoga tradition of the time (third century C.E.), and as the collaboration between Yogācāra and Tantra became more intense over the next few centuries, the persona of at least the Yogācāra practitioners came to resemble more that of the Indian yogi than that of the Buddhist monk.

It also seems a reasonable speculation that the popularity of Buddhism in China and later in Tibet had a lot to do with its reputation as a religion of magic and mystery, a trend fueled more than anything else by Yogācāra's collaboration with Tantra. Today, the Vajrayāna Buddhism of Tibet is indistinct from its self-perception as Tantric Buddhism, meaning it is esoteric and practice-oriented. The variety of rituals and practices in Tibetan Buddhism testify both to its centuries-old collaboration with Yoga and to its ancestry in the Indo-Tibetan Buddhism. The practices of Tantric Buddhism make it almost impossible to put a separation point between "Yoga" and "Buddhism" in that tradition.

The enduring connection of yogic practices with magic and mystery has meant that at the folk level in all the countries of East and North Asia, Buddhism has been considered a religion of magic and mystery. Its philosophical doctrines may be of interest to a few elite, but for the majority of people in these countries Buddhism and Yoga, that is, magical powers, remain inseparable. Indeed, one of the first Western travelers to Tibet in the early years of the twentieth century, Alexandra David-Neel (1868–1969), captured the imagination of the West through her description of Tibet as the land of magic and mystery.

The word *Yoga* is used freely and casually in Tibetan Buddhism as a testament to its self-perception that its yogic practices are but a continuation of the paradigm according to which the historical Śākyamuni Buddha lived his own life. Practices such as doing meditation in isolated caves for months and years are not only encouraged but also required of high lamas. These practices are not the self-mortification practices of the śramaṇa culture of the Buddha's time but entail visualizations of named deities that may be described by the practitioner in terms almost identical with those used by a yogi in ancient India of pre-Buddhist times.

What this means for the contemporary practitioner of "Buddhism" (or mindfulness) or "Yoga" is that there's a need to align oneself with the worldviews of these traditions if one is to go beyond the habits of consuming desires and to use these traditions as consumer items. Of course, one can always say that one does not give a hoot about their original intention or worldviews. That would be a fair position if one is participating in it as a consumer without any claims about "spirituality." But if any such claims are made, then the issues of original intention and contexts can become quite vexing.

10

A TWISTED STORY

JILL SATTERFIELD

A SPIRITUAL SEARCH usually begins with the recognition of some sort of suffering, whether physical, emotional, or mental. Finding an end to suffering was the Buddha's original quest twenty-five hundred years ago, and the object of that quest continues to propel people into Yoga studios, meditation centers, and various other spiritual homes.

Seeking an end to suffering can also imply a willingness to look at and consider the causes of suffering, and an understanding of impermanence. Those fortunate enough to stumble across the Buddha's teachings will discover that there is already a diagnosis, prescription, course of action, and the possibility of total recovery from what ails us—or, what we "think" might ail us: a journey of discovery in its own right.

For me, the intertwining of Buddhism and Yoga arose organically as a literal twisting and untwisting that occurred in my physical body. At twenty years old, I was struck with searing pain. I was in art school in New York City at the time, and had been in fact debating with my fellow students earlier in the month about whether or not—since I had grown up in a nice home, with a loving family—I had suffered enough to create really good art. It was an ironic karmic twist that physical agony would suddenly be offered as a way of suffering for my art, or for anything really.

I'd had no prior experience with serious pain, so I did as I'd been taught to do: "rise above and ignore." After several months, I finally had to surrender (as I viewed it at the time) and seek medical help. I found a doctor I thought would be able to determine the cause of the pain and know immediately how to fix it.

At our first meeting, I suspected that this doctor didn't truly believe me when I tried to describe the amount of pain I was in. He repeatedly commented on how healthy I appeared, how pretty I looked. He was dismissive and haughty, and said he couldn't find any organic cause for the symptoms I described. Not knowing what else to do, however, I continued to see him, reiterating the same complaints every time, even bringing him a drawing of myself and all the places I felt the pain. I think he finally arranged to have me undergo exploratory surgery simply in order to end my visits.

The surgery revealed that an ovary had become attached to part of my large intestine. The organs were separated and I was assured that all would be well after a brief period of rest. However, all was not well and I continued to experience excruciating, chronic pain. I returned to this doctor again and again until he finally announced that the pain must be in my mind: he could see nothing else causing it. "If it's in my mind," I asked him, having no idea that I was foreshadowing a solution I would later find for myself, "then what can I do about my mind?" He was not amused.

Over the next several years I went from one specialist to another, continually thinking, "This one will save me," "This next one will be able to fix me," "This new person surely has to have the answers." I underwent what felt like every test known to medical science, and yet no one could determine the reason for my continued pain. Over and over, my hopes were shattered. Over and over, it was suggested that the pain was a "phantom," a "figment of my overactive imagination," a "female problem": just take two of these, five of something else, and go away—we can't help you.

In the meantime, I accidentally started taking a Yoga class. It was called "movement," but it was unlike any other movement class I had taken, so I asked the teacher what kind of movement it was and she whispered, "Yoga." I was so immediately drawn to the experiences I had in her class that I took as many classes as I could find, which in the late seventies wasn't so easy. I moved an hour north of New York City, so it was even more challenging to find classes, but fortunately I found some excellent Iyengar-trained teachers.

I started practicing Yoga at home, from a Sivananda book that had sequences in it. I liked practicing alone, for several reasons. Alone, I didn't feel the need to impress anyone—no matter how hard I tried to get around it, I still worked a bit more in a pose when others were in the room. I often felt emotional in poses as well, and wanted to have the option of stopping and crying if I needed to, which I wasn't at all comfortable about doing in front of others. Moreover, the teacher whose class I attended most frequently was constantly emphasizing the, as yet to my mind unsupported, fact of the healing effects of Yoga. Her pronouncements made me feel even more isolated in my illness and, along with years of being marginalized by doctors, made me feel like I was the only person in a Yoga class who wasn't well—this situation didn't exactly fill me with hope. This feeling of being (unfortunately) unique and beyond repair would later materialize, surprisingly, as a magnificent gift for empathy that I would later appreciate as a teacher.

I continued practicing Yoga anyway, simply because I liked it rather than because I thought it would save or heal me. In fact, I also continued to experience constant pain. My humiliating past encounters with doctors kept me as far away from them as possible for about three years, until I couldn't stay away any longer. I went to a well-respected gynecologist at Johns Hopkins University Hospital in Maryland. After hearing my story, he sent me in for another exploratory surgery. This was my fifth exploratory surgery. He found another cause for my pain: ovarian cysts. He removed part of each ovary, and genuinely thought that would be the end of my problems. However, after a lengthy recovery of a month in bed, I was still in tremendous pain.

A New Twist

More years went by—eight since the first time I'd sought medical help. I tried different doctors, undergoing a variety of new tests, none of which shed any light on the cause of my pain. All the "rising above" had been exhausting. The painkillers only made me dull, and I was losing my ability to be joyful. I became difficult to be around: for example, I would feel a surge of intense, unexpected pain in the middle of a party or a dinner, which would render me speechless or streaming tears. I felt guilty about sounding like a broken record—and about being just plain broken. I was in my late twenties and I felt robbed of any semblance of a normal life.

Finally, out of complete desperation and exasperation, I sought out a local surgeon and asked him if he would open me up once again. In order to get him to agree, I convinced him that the pain was truly organic and that I couldn't continue to live with it anymore. He looked around a bit more than previous doctors, and found yet another cause for the pain—one that was truly bizarre. I had always thought that I was different: first because of the natural development of my delusional ego, then as an artist, then as someone in chronic pain, so in an odd way I felt justified about feeling so special! My large intestine had knotted, twisted, and traveled all the way up to my heart, taking the appendix along with it and herniating my diaphragm along the way. Finally I was healed, I was saved—or at least, I had a cause for what pained me.

After six weeks of bed rest I was finally able to walk around, but since I had an incision that ran from my pubic bone to my navel, I could barely lift a plate full of food. I was convinced, though, that this time I would eventually become pain free and back to "normal."

Three more years went by. Although I was in pain most of the time, I kept "a stiff upper lip," would "rise above and ignore," and "put a smile on my face" as I'd been taught as a child. Most people were never aware of the extent of my discomfort. I became proficient at hiding it and not talking about it. Frankly, I even bored myself with my "pain story" and its chapters full of complaints.

In addition to practicing Yoga, I also tried a variety of alternative practitioners. I made appointments with people who charged me a substantial amount of money to wave a wand around my head and give me odd-looking concoctions to boil and ingest. Some suggested affirmations for me; others recommended books about powerful women to read, suggesting I needed some sort of heroine to relate to. I'd never been into "voodoo" practices per se, but I was open to anything at that point.

My patience with nonscientific methods eventually wore thin, and my tolerance had holes in it at that point, so I decided to go to the Yale Pain Clinic. Surely, they would be able to help me at least manage the pain. I booked an appointment and waited a month with optimistic anticipation for the day to arrive. I drove up to New Haven with a tremendous load of blind faith that someone at Yale would finally, finally help me.

Unfortunately, the solutions they offered were more excruciating to hear about than was my experience of the physical pain itself. Surgeons could perform a nerve block so that I didn't register any sensation in the right side of my pelvis, but the surgery was accompanied by incredibly high risks. Because the area to be operated on was close to my spine, the surgery could possibly paralyze me. There was also a small chance that the operation could put me into a coma. I never asked how or why: just hearing that was enough to compel me to get up and leave.

I walked out to my car defeated and deflated. I cried so hard that the parking-lot attendant made me wait until I had calmed down before he would let me exit the lot. I pulled myself together sufficiently to leave, but cried my way home. The hour-long drive became a cathartic experience, though, because halfway home I made a vow: that I would help myself get well, I would figure this out on my own, I finally got it that I couldn't rely on anyone else to help me. I had to help myself.

Straightening Up My Home/Body

I suppose I had the option of giving up, but it didn't occur to me. Instead, I began to do some research. This was pre-Internet, so libraries and bookstores became my second home. I had an intuition that food could help me, as I had a difficult time digesting, so I looked into the healing properties of food. I studied the area of my body that wasn't working properly—the intestinal tract. I learned how it functioned optimally, what it looked like and where it was located (or relocated, in my case). I studied anatomy—enough to have a good idea of where organs and glands were and what their functions consisted of. I learned about muscles by looking them up in *Grey's Anatomy,* then trying to sense them while moving around in a Yoga pose. Reading that the Buddha recommended sitting, standing, walking, and lying down as postures suitable for meditation, I began to see my āsana practice as a combination of those four choices, with an understanding of impermanence and relative reality found in his *Satipaṭṭhāna Sutta:*

> A monk reflects on this very body from the soles of the feet on up, from the crown of the head on down, surrounded by skin and full of various kinds of unclean things: "In this body there are head hairs, body hairs, nails, teeth, skin, flesh, tendons, bones, bone marrow, kidneys, heart, liver, pleura, spleen, lungs, large intestines, small intestines, gorge, feces, bile, phlegm, pus, blood, sweat, fat, tears, skin-oil, saliva, mucus, fluid in the joints, urine."[1]

This graphic and simple description of a body was exactly what I needed to see my body as just a body, and work with observing it as such.

Rather than just question why practicing Yoga wasn't healing my body, I was now compelled to find out why not. Was I missing something? I began to read about Yoga's origins and its healing potential. I had no idea that there were so many different ways to practice Yoga, or that Hatha was only a small component of a much larger field of physical, philosophical, and spiritual disciplines. This information came at just the right time to give me some hope that maybe I just hadn't found the best way to practice yet. I was especially inspired by this passage from B. K. S. Iyengar's *Light on Yoga:*

> Where does the body end and the mind begin? They cannot be divided as they are inter-related and but different aspects of the same all-pervading divine consciousness.[2]

I had intuited the mind-body connection, but to read a statement from such a well-respected teacher gave me the confidence I needed, not only to continue my search for understanding the connection of body and mind but to unleash the power of utilizing the connection. A quote from Pantañjali offered another source of both inspiration and hope:

> Through faith, which will give sufficient energy to achieve success against all odds, direction will be maintained. The realization of the goal of Yoga is a matter of time.[3]

I was very willing and able to give myself the time to practice and beat the odds.

I also had this seemingly radical notion that perhaps I should consider that the pain could simply be in my mind at this point; and if that were the case, what could I do about it? I realized that I knew little about my own mind, and I knew that my mind mattered.

> We have to go through the process of sitting down and examining the mind and examining our experience to see what is really going on.[4]

Although I hadn't read this quote by Kalu Rinpoche at the time, I intuited the necessity of examination as one of the best ways of working with my situation. I wasn't exactly sure how to go about getting to know my mind, but I did know that my mind was racing and anxious, and I had heard a lot about meditation calming the mind, so I found a local meditation group. I loved the sitting practice, but not, as it turned out, for the reason I initially went. I found myself feeling extremely high and ecstatic while meditating. I wasn't getting to know my mind, but leaving it and my body behind. Although the experience was terrifically pleasant, I was all over the place mentally. I knew even then that I needed to stay grounded in order to understand my mind, so I looked for another tradition that might help me do that.

Sitting Straight

On the advice of a friend, I decided to explore Vipassanā meditation. I knew I needed to immerse myself, so I jumped right into a ten-day retreat led by students of S. N. Goenka. This was the first time in my life that I'd committed myself to sit still with any and all sensations, emotions, and thoughts. I practiced their remarkable body-scanning technique, which I continue to utilize as a way of becoming meticulously aware of my entire physical being. Beginning at the crown of the head, you linger there until you feel a sensation, and then proceed a quarter of an inch either to one side or down, moving slowly along your entire body. Though such a minute investigation can literally take hours, bringing the mind so closely into its physical realm and investigating sensations in such a microcosmic way affords you the opportunity to get to know your body extremely well. Upon practicing this technique for the first time, I felt as if a veil had been lifted: I could recognize the distinction between what was real and what was imagined, as well as the impermanence of both states of mind. In other words, I could stay in my mind and lose feeling of my body, which was imagined, and I could also stay with the sensations in my body and witness them arise, change, and fade, which was very real.

I also noticed that I wouldn't "die" if I remained consciously aware of uncomfortable feelings—and as someone brought up to deny any "negative" feelings, this was, in itself, an enormous accomplishment. I had been deeply programmed to move away from discomfort of any kind, whether physical or emotional. I had no idea how hard it was to watch my breath after I got bored or to feel emotional pain for more than a brief second. But to my surprise I did it. I felt like a scientist, able to see how my mind worked and how my body would process my mind. When my mind was spacious and quiet, the pain in my body became more of a decoration than a declaration. Both of my practices completely enhanced the other. My body became a body, not just mine. My mind became more fascinating—not so heavy and serious. After every meditation retreat—and I attended several in quick succession over the next seven years—I felt lighter and more at ease with what is. The Buddha suggested four postures suitable for meditation—seated, standing, lying down, and walking. I stretched this a bit to mean to mean that practicing a Yoga posture became just another shape in which to meditate. Being in my body, then, became a doorway to being in the present moment and not flying far, far away.

Sometimes while practicing poses, it was as if I were reliving drug-enhanced experiences. I began traveling deeply inside my body like Alice down the rabbit hole, into a world of dark spaces as well as colorful designs. I could wander around inside using my breath as a guide, and discover which areas needed attention and care and which ones offered a certain kind of delight—a sparkling, vibratory experience. I played around, imagining tossing fairy dust into my veins and making my intestines sparkle. I visualized my pelvis as a giant glass bowl with brightly colored flower petals at the base. With my breath I would swirl the petals around and around the bowl, bringing vibrancy back, if only in my imagination. What I didn't know at the time was that it wasn't simply a case of engaging my imagination: my body was physically being healed at the same time, without my conscious awareness.

Six months later I ventured over to the Insight Meditation Society, where I met my first and present teacher, Ajahn Amaro. One significant technique I learned early on from him was the art of contemplation. His instructions were so simple and clear. Quiet the mind and choose a subject, the bigger the better, such as "mother." Drop the "subject" into the quiet lake of the mind and just wait to see what bubbles up. Mom, Mommy, Mum, and so on—repeat the words, the ideas, and wait to see what associations arise. I would practice this type of contemplation to uncover emotional patterns caught in my body, imagining my body as my house. I scanned my body as if it were a property with which I was becoming reacquainted and seeing more clearly, like coming home from a trip away. I would imagine where I stored my childhood memories, and what that particular area of my body felt like; where my parents stayed when they came for "a visit," where I needed "repair," where the house was the darkest and where it held the most light.

This type of creative contemplation provided me with intuition about my emotional body, and once again how my body processed my mind. Pursuing this link gave me a key to what I believe was a turning point in healing my body. I harnessed the power of my own mind to locate areas that needed attention and care, areas that I needed to "clean and air out," problems I might need to actually talk through with someone else (as in parent-related issues), where I needed to bring in more light—which, in my mind, meant awareness. At this point I was convinced I had the power to help myself heal.

I would position myself in a Yoga pose that opened that particular area and I would wait for my eyes to adjust to the darkened space—just resting my mind. It was as if I became my own best friend: the friend as a witness to the stories my body needed to tell, who stayed no matter what came up, who never made me feel embarrassed or small, who believed everything I said.

Mostly while on retreat, which I began doing five or six times a year, I would intentionally imagine peristalsis over and over again. I started this visualization at the beginning of the large intestine, and worked my way down to the end—a kind of variation on the Goenka body scan I had learned on my first retreat. I coaxed my body over and over to remember what it was like to work normally, as normally as when I was a child, before the problems began. I yearned to simply reawaken it from its slumber by reintroducing the patterns of movement it once had had.

Eventually I was no longer afraid to sit with discomfort. I could experience pain as sensation as well as a uniquely changeable experience that wasn't always unpleasant. Initially, just allowing the pain to be, without moving my mind away from it or trying to transform it, was a challenge. Eventually, though, I was able to view pain as a sensation—neither comfortable nor uncomfortable, that simply arose and changed.

I spent one ten-day retreat just focusing in on and dissecting an entire area of pain—using the pain as the support for my practice rather my breath. The painful area was huge and emotionally overwhelming—it usually encompassed the entire right side of my pelvis, often moving into my right leg. But when I stayed with that single sensation, it gradually broke into many smaller ones, and I began to distinguish between them—some felt like a tickle or tingling, for instance. I found that when I stayed with each sensation, I could eventually locate the nadir of the pain. Through this process of dissection, the pain lost its ability to frighten me—by literally shrinking. Even though freedom from intense pain might happen for only moments at a time, if I looked pain directly in the face, it lost its power to overwhelm me, and my body could relax around it. I felt larger than the pain, like a person gaining her full personality back, not to be labeled or to only relate to myself as a person in pain. When one becomes overly identified with something like pain or illness, it can narrow and constrict life. I felt as though I'd opened an aperture and allowed my view to widen. I returned to being more than just a person in pain.

As the Twist Turned

After imagining my intestines waking up and working normally time and time again, they actually began to work on their own. I was ecstatic; I was returning to normal! This turn of events totally shocked the doctors I told, as they had repeatedly insisted that there was no way to retrigger peristalsis: it was a part of the autonomic nervous system and, like the breath, functioned without our conscious control. Fortunately, being a yogi and practicing prāṇāyāma, I was brazen enough to think I might have the same control over peristalsis, which is what actually happened. A quote by Bokar Rinpoche, from *The Profound Wisdom of the Heart Sūtra,* gave me the confidence to retrain not only my mind but my body as well:

> We should not forget that the mind, whatever turn that we want to give it, is very flexible. To the extent that we train ourselves, we create a habit and the mind accepts the crease that we give it.[5]

Once in a while I could actually feel my intestines move and unwind: a surreal experience, and one that at first I thought I was imagining. Once, though, I looked down at my abdomen and saw it actually move as I felt something wriggling around. This would only happen when I was concentrated with particular effort on the area and was imagining moving a tingling feeling through my pelvis. As my practices were weaving together, my body was literally unwinding.

I knew for certain that my mind was moving my body, moving inside of my body, motivating my body. The unknotting of my mind created the spacious atmosphere for the intestines and the muscular area around them to do the same. The physical, energetic, seen, and unseen were now living compatibly and consciously in my home/body. This reconciliation was seven years in the making—getting to know my mind, body, and heart to the degree that they could communicate intimately.

Meeting Tibetan Buddhist meditation masters facilitated this process tremendously. After seven years of Vipassana retreats, I attended a Tibetan Buddhist meditation retreat, and became close to several teachers. One teacher loved to hear the details of my recent healing, and urged me to teach what I had discovered. He also gently pressed me to tell my story of healing, saying it might help others, but it took me a good five years to share this story with anyone without feeling embarrassed by the oddity of it. Mingyur Rinpoche, my current teacher, taught me a great deal about loving-kindness and compassion, which has enabled me to continue to heal on an emotional level in addition to the physical—and the two are completely intertwined. After the pain began to subside, I was able to investigate the area of my pelvis emotionally and to slowly accept some of the stories it held about being hurt or disappointed as a young child. I had insights about these memories on silent retreats, but it was through compassion for myself that I was able to forgive others and myself for what had hurt me.

I had been searching for someone to save me, thinking that others might know more about my mind-body than I did. With respect to the physical positioning of my intestines, it turned out I did indeed need external help, but all other aspects of help needed to be of my own devising. The drawing I had brought to that very first doctor in New York resurfaced during a move I made ten years ago. It turned out that the points of pain I had drawn along various parts of my body were the meridian lines for the large intestine. Many of the drawings I'd made during those years of chronic pain look now like twisted intestines, and mini-implosions. Some of the visualizations that I thought I had made up have been found in books describing Tibetan tantric techniques, and have been called by one of my teachers "bliss." Apparently I had, without knowing it, tapped into a number of ancient traditions. I now teach from this vantage point: that we can know a great deal more about ourselves than we have been led in our culture to believe, and that when it comes to utilizing the power of our minds, we are only at the beginning.

Straight to the Heart

I'm grateful for all of these experiences, which I truly never thought I would be able to have the luxury of saying. Having had something as stubborn and persistent a teacher as pain presented me with a vessel (my body) from which I found compassion and resolve. My illness brought interdependence to the forefront of my consciousness (ironically even while part of my intestine traveled to meet my heart), that my mind is indeed connected to my body, that I am not the separate entity I first believed myself to be, that we all share the common goal of happiness.

The paths of Yoga and Buddhism intertwined without any type of manipulation on my part. For once, I didn't have to work so hard to twist or untwist, or take care of any details; the connection was organic. Following the Buddha's teachings have inspired me to help others help themselves, to assist others to get to know their own mind, body, and heart a bit better, and to take positive action armed with the best information available.

Yoga postures can be a doorway into the mind, an invitation to witness our minds through the physical entrance that most of us can relate to. When the body becomes the conscious home for the mind, and is able to fully inhabit its form, this connection becomes an invitation to experience emptiness. This experience allows us to loosen the grip of ego so that we may relate to the body as just a body, the mind as just a mind, and embrace experientially the interconnectedness of life—and the compassion that naturally blooms from this realization.

As I entered into Buddhism through the physical door, I have invited many others to do the same through the postures of Yoga and mindfulness of the body. For many of us, it is easier to relate to the body than to the mind—so the practice of mindfulness in the body is a practical means for seeing the mind without feeling overwhelmed by a sitting meditation practice. It can be an organic introduction to how this body works, feels, and "wears" the mind. The mind can be seen as the inhabitant of the "house," the one that can rearrange the furniture, open the windows, clean the closets. Often a Yoga practice imbued with awareness empowers others to take further skillful and conscious action to make positive choices in their lives. I have seen this over the twenty years I have been teaching Yoga and meditation, and am especially passionate about working with those who normally wouldn't have the opportunity to practice these traditions, or who might feel alone in their search for health and healing.

Bound Together

Feeling so alone in my illness, so marginalized and misunderstood, became the seed of intention that has propelled me to help anyone I could not to have to feel the same way. My tools are my practices and, most importantly, my experiences. I've sought out ways of bringing the Buddhist view and the postures of Yoga into places where people wouldn't normally have the opportunity to practice them, and have developed the Social Action Teacher Training to train teachers to work with at-risk youth and adults, people in recovery from substances, and those living in chronic pain and with illnesses. This work allows me to share my story, give hope, and offer practical means to those in need who would not be likely to wander into a Yoga studio or meditation center. The goal is to serve others, but where do we start? We have to start with ourselves. "If I am going to serve you, I have to start with myself, by improving my attitude and actions to make myself a good servant for you, to make myself a proper tool to serve you,"[6] said Tulku Thondup, and this is exactly what our intention is. Get to now your own mind, body, and heart, and you have a tremendous amount of insight and information to share with others so that they may do the same.

The Dalai Lama has said that it's easier to meditate than to actually do things for others, and that we should all seize opportunities to take action and do something skillful in society. I couldn't agree more. Our practices, once matured, organically bloom into the desire to help others help themselves, and there are plenty of people to help in the world. I have chosen to take steps in my local community by training teachers to venture into populations where the benefits of our practices may not be known or available. My private pain has become my public announcement, and will hopefully reach many, many others with hope, choice, and the desire to help one another. It is my hope that American Buddhism will continue to flourish with integrity and courage—to be woven deeply into the fabric of our culture in a practical and meaningful way.

11

MINDFULNESS YOGA

FRANK JUDE BOCCIO

FOR THE VAST majority of practitioners and nonpractitioners alike, Yoga has become reduced to, and synonymous with, the postures and movements of Hatha Yoga. An article recently published in a respected Yoga magazine included the following statement: "Each day began with Yoga and ended with meditation." Yet for most of its history, meditation has been an essential aspect of authentic Yoga practice, and such statements evince a fundamental misunderstanding with Yoga understood as relating to the body and meditation being purely mental. However, deeper investigation reveals the inaccuracy of such a view. Much of the "work" of meditation involves how we experience the body, particularly our reactivity to experience. And when practicing postures, we learn to deal with the mind's commentary, which creates story lines and judgments, leans toward the future or the past, grasps after the pleasant, and pushes away the unpleasant—exactly what we deal with in meditation!

Yoga's seedbed lies over four thousand years ago with the Indus/ Sarasvatī civilization of northwest India. The word *Yoga* comes from the root *yuj,* meaning to "yoke or to harness," and by extension has come to signify both spiritual endeavor, especially the disciplining of the mind and the senses, and the state of integration. Interestingly, the Latin root of the word *religion*—*religio*—means "to tie or bind back." Free of institutional forms and meanings, the similar definition of these two words points to the essentially religious purpose of all Yoga practice. As found in the *Vedas,* the oldest of the sacred scriptures of Hinduism, a kind of proto-Yoga seems to have been the practice of disciplined, meditative focusing on the proper performance of elaborate sacrificial rituals.

Then, from around 1500 to 1000 B.C.E., a countercultural movement arose, transforming this outwardly focused ritualized system into a more internalized form of spiritual practice replete with esoteric teachings that were gradually compiled into the *Upaniṣads*. It was here that we find teachings and practices recognizable as "Yoga." The word *Upaniṣad* means "sitting down near" (as one does when studying with one's teacher), pointing to the fact that Upaniṣadic teachings were delivered directly from teacher to student by word of mouth. The teacher-student relationship remains of great importance for the direct transmission of yogic wisdom and experience.

As such, Yoga is the generic name for the various Indian philosophies and practices Georg Feuerstein calls "the psychospiritual technology specific to the great civilization of India,"[1] the purpose of which is to liberate the practitioner from the existential human situation of duḥkha. Out of this greater Yoga tradition emerged the three major yogic cultural complexes of India: Hinduism, Buddhism, and Jainism.

I stress this dynamic process because all too often Yoga is spoken of as if it were some monolithic, homogenous entity when in fact the views and practices vary from school to school, often even contradicting one another. Most are nondual, but there are also dualistic schools as well as every imaginable viewpoint in between! When I speak of Yoga (with a capital Y), I am referring to the ocean of yogic teachings that predate and permeate Hinduism, Buddhism, and Jainism, representing a multitude of paths, views, philosophical contexts, and apparently different goals, although each school agrees upon the need to address, transcend, or resolve the human situation of duḥkha.

Given this context, it should be obvious that I view Buddhism as a bona fide child of the Yoga tradition, with the Buddha's teachings, known as Buddhadharma, completely yogic in purpose, intent, and methodology. The Four Noble Truths and Eightfold Path offer a complete and coherent model of yogic theory and practice. In fact, it is one of the earliest such models, predating Patañjali's *Yoga Sūtra* by over five hundred years. Like all authentic Yoga, it is mokṣa-śāstra, a liberation teaching designed to free us from duḥkha.

In referring to Patañjali's teachings, I use the terms *classical Yoga* and *Rāja Yoga*. Classical Yoga is considered one of the six "orthodox" schools of Indian philosophy, considered "orthodox" because they share a common belief in the *Vedas* as revealed knowledge. It is important to remember that these schools evolved over time, often centuries after their alleged "founders." Many scholars today debate whether the understandings of later commentators truly reflect the original teaching of Patañjali.

With the term *Hatha Yoga,* I refer to the relatively recent form of yogic practice utilizing the familiar postures (āsanas) as well as breathing practices (prāṇāyāma) that in contemporary times have become synonymous with Yoga. This form of Yoga practice has its roots in the Tantra Yoga movement that influenced both Hindu and Buddhist Yoga traditions. While the āsanas of Hatha Yoga are what most Westerners are familiar with as Yoga, such postures were developed rather late in the history of the Yoga tradition. For most of Yoga's history, practice meant meditation, chanting, selfless service, and study. This broader understanding of Yoga makes it clear that whenever a Buddhist takes her seat in the meditation hall, she is practicing Yoga.

However, when I began to study and practice both Hatha Yoga and Zen Buddhism in the mid-1970s, it was common to be told by Zen teachers that "sitting" was all one needed. Zazen was the be-all and end-all of practice, and if one practiced assiduously enough, nothing else was necessary—certainly *not* (Hatha) Yoga! Despite the ruin of many a knee, most teachers were pretty firm in this blanket condemnation. To those at the zendo where I practiced, yogis were bliss addicts, in complete denial of duḥkha—the existence of suffering—and they looked askance at my dedication to Hatha Yoga practice.

Meanwhile, at the ashram where I practiced Hatha Yoga, I was repeatedly told that Hatha Yoga is a complete spiritual discipline and that posture practice was preparatory to meditation—but we never meditated in class! As for my interest in Zen Buddhism, as far as those yogis were concerned, there couldn't be a more dour, joyless, lot than Zen students, sitting stock-still in the severe, colorless zendo, "obsessed" with suffering.

This mutual distrust between the practitioners of Hatha Yoga and Zen was based on the common misunderstanding of the cultural affinities between Yoga and Buddhism. Yet from the start I knew—and confirmed in my own experience—that these practices had much to offer each other. Over the past three decades, many Buddhist meditators (including Zen students!) have been drawn to Hatha Yoga for the ease and strength it can bring to the body, while many Hatha yogis have turned to Buddhist meditation for the deepening of awareness, insight, and equanimity it can cultivate.

While this "complementary" approach has much to offer, I've found that a deeper, more integrated, comprehensive approach is possible. The complementary approach still looks at Yoga and Buddhism (represented as meditation) as different, with Yoga being about the body, and Buddhism (and meditation generally) being about the mind. Yet, as shown above, this is an inaccurate view!

In an early discourse, the Buddha is asked if it is possible, by traveling, to know, see, or to reach the end of the world, where one does not suffer. He responds by saying that it is not possible to reach such a place of peace by traveling. "However, I say that without having reached the end of the world there is no making an end to suffering. It is, friend, in just this fathom-high body endowed with perception and mind that I make known the world, its arising and cessation, and the way leading to the cessation of the world."[2] The Buddha could not have more clearly stated that it is with the exploration of our bodily experience, where we so often find discomfort, pain, and suffering, that we can also find peace and liberation.

So while things have changed since the seventies, I believe they haven't changed enough. The primary cause of the false distinction between Yoga and Buddhadharma is the historical anomaly that the physical aspect of Hatha Yoga, the āsanas, first caught the attention of Western students. For many, the great diversity of the Yoga tradition was reduced to the mere physical performance of the postures and movements of Hatha Yoga. But the primary meaning of the word *Yoga* as "to yoke" is descriptive of what we do when we restrain our attention from wandering when sitting in meditation. We "yoke" our attention to our object of meditation.

Originally, the prime activity of the yogi was to sit in meditation. The Sanskrit word for the seat he took was "ās" (pronounced with a broad *ah* sound, "ahs"). The proper and natural posture of the body in sitting meditation is called āsana, defined by the second-century Indian sage Patañjali in the *Yoga Sūtra,* the foundational text of classical Yoga, as that posture that is both "stable and easeful,"[3] accompanied by "the relaxation of effort and the revealing of the body and the infinite universe as indivisible."[4] When this state is attained, "one is no longer disturbed by the play of opposites."[5]

The other meaning of the word *Yoga*—"union"—refers to the integration of body, breath, and mind in each moment, and to the dropping away of the sense of separation between "self" as subject of experience and "other" as object of experience. Whenever this state of embodied integration manifests—whether one is sitting, walking, cutting carrots, or changing diapers—*there* is Yoga.

When sitting, we enter intimately into the experience of the body. Yet how can we experience the "stability and ease" these great teachers speak of when our bodies are so often filled with tension, pain, or self-deprecation? How can we become truly intimate with our physical bodies and become liberated from our clinging identification with the body as "me" or "mine," and access that deep peace, realizing the indivisibility of the body and the infinite universe?

As for many who come to spiritual practice, these kinds of questions, and the situation in which they arose, motivated me to begin practicing Yoga. It is what yogis call duḥkha. This Sanskrit word, most commonly translated as "suffering," "dissatisfaction," "stress," "anguish," "discontentment," "unease," "affliction," and "anxiety," literally means "bad space," understood at the time of the Buddha to describe a misaligned axle, that is to say, a wheel whose axle is not centered. Imagine an oxcart rolling along a rutted dirt road with a misaligned axle. It would undoubtedly be a jarring, uncomfortable ride! Or imagine a ceramic wheel. Anyone who's attempted to work clay with a misaligned wheel knows the difficulty of trying to create something beautiful and useful under such conditions. The Buddha emphasizes that when we are not aligned with reality, when not in balance with the truth of the present moment, we are in for a difficult ride through life. We will have a challenging time trying to live a lovely and useful life. Ultimately, duḥkha can be described as that sense of "something's not right," that something's missing, the feeling of alienation that drives us to search in myriad places for that which we seem to lack: connection, wholeness, freedom from this pervasive sense of discontent.

The Buddha studied with two Yoga masters, Ālāro Kālāmo and Uddako Rāmaputto, attaining the highest states of concentration taught at that time. However, the Buddha felt that such states were not the full liberation of nirvāṇa. He said that in such states "there is liberation from form and formlessness, (but) there is still something left over—the thing that has been liberated from them, a watcher. As long as such a watcher remains, though one may momentarily be secluded from the cycle of suffering, the watcher remains as a seed of rebirth."[6] Once samādhi ends and situational conditions change, "rebirth takes place again." He adds, "No matter how profound the absorption, after a short time I get caught up again in the world of the senses. The basic causes and conditions for rebirth have not been extinguished! Complete liberation has not been achieved!"[7]

When first told the story of the Buddha's life, I was led to believe that in leaving his teachers he rejected Yoga, but now I see that while he refuted his teachers' interpretation of the meditative states they taught as being liberation, he did not turn his back on the technology of Yoga. What the Buddha rejected was the idea of a separate Self or Subject that, as he noted, would only become the seed for "rebirth." This understanding, by the way, need not be taken metaphysically. The rebirth of a sense of self, what Patañjali calls asmitā, is what happens in each moment of reactivity; the cycle of birth, aging, passing away, and rebirth refers to the sense of a separate self that arises in reaction to events and situations. This is what the Buddha means when he says the world "arises and ceases" in this fathom-long body.

The Buddha, as a consummate yogi, refused to accept anyone else's metaphysics, interpretations, or dogma, relying on his own direct experience. While he refuted the mainstream metaphysics of Vedic-based Yoga teachings, his own teaching and practice are firmly rooted in the broader Yoga tradition. While the Buddha taught a variety of practices, perhaps it's his emphasis on mindfulness, and methods to cultivate it, that has had the greatest impact. The Pali word *sati* (Skt: smṛti), most often translated as "mindfulness" or "awareness," relates to memory and the word for remembering. To "re-member" is to "re-collect," to bring together all the seemingly disparate aspects of our experience into an integrated whole. In this way, remembering is synonymous with the definition of Yoga. Whenever we see our mind wandering from the intimate, immediate, spontaneous, and obvious experience at hand, we remember to come back—to just this, right here, right now, using the breath as the yoke.

In the *Bhaddekaratta Sutta,* the Buddha taught, "Looking deeply at life as it is in the very here and now, the practitioner dwells in stability and freedom."[8] In both the *Ānāpānasati Sutta* (Awareness of Breathing), and the *Satipaṭṭhāna Sutta* (The Foundation of Mindfulness), the

Buddha instructs us to observe the breath, gradually extending our awareness to include the whole body. He says the practitioner should be aware of the movements and positions of the body while standing, walking, sitting, or lying down, while bending over or stretching one's limbs, and notes that nothing is excluded from mindfulness, including such activities as eating, drinking, dressing, urinating, and defecating. No aspect of our lived experience lies outside of practice. Ideally, there is no separation between "formal" practice and the rest of our lives. This is not practice as preparation, but practice as vocation.

The applicability of this teaching for practicing Hatha Yoga is obvious. When we combine awareness of breathing with āsana practice, we can observe how movement affects the breath and how the breath affects the body. We become aware of habitual patterns of reactivity. For instance, do you hold your breath when reaching out with your arms into a deep stretch? Do you unnecessarily tense muscles not involved with the movement you are making? Do you compare one side of the body with the other? When engaged in repetitive movements, does your mind wander? In maintaining a posture, can you see the constant changing phenomena, or do you concretize the experience, reifying the changing phenomena into a static entity that you then either grasp after or resist, depending on whether you find it pleasant or unpleasant?

For years I practiced the postures and movements of Hatha Yoga as a complement to my mindfulness meditation practice. I benefited greatly from the physical practice—greater flexibility and ease within the body, more balanced energy, better respiratory efficiency—and experienced the more subtle benefits of greater body awareness and a settling of the mind that helped prepare me for sitting meditation.

But on retreat with Thich Nhat Hanh where he presented the Four Foundations of Mindfulness, a core meditation practice taught by the Buddha, I was led to a deeper, more integrated, comprehensive way of practicing. Following the Four Foundations of Mindfulness, the practice of postures becomes much more than merely preparation for meditation. With the Four Foundations, āsana practice becomes a fully authentic mindfulness practice, in essence no different from sitting or walking meditation. On Vipassanā retreats, sessions of sitting meditation are alternated with equal-length sessions of walking meditation. While sitting may seem central to the practice, one doesn't walk in order to prepare for it. Walking is simply another way of practicing mindfulness, just as eating or work practice are conceived as mindfulness practices. Likewise, āsana practice need not be conceptualized as a complement or preliminary to sitting. It's simply another way to practice mindfulness.

This is the practice of Mindfulness Yoga, not mindful Yoga. The distinction is clear. With the term *mindful Yoga*, an adjective modifies a noun while with Mindfulness Yoga the whole term is a proper noun. It's the difference between saying, "Let's practice Triangle mindfully" and "Let's practice mindfulness through the form of Triangle." In the first example, the priority is the āsana to which you add the quality of mindfully practicing it, while in the second case the priority is the cultivation of mindfulness and the āsana is the vehicle for such cultivation. The practice of mindfulness, the Buddha assures us, "gives rise to understanding and liberation of the mind."

The Four Foundations of Mindfulness include body, feelings, mind, and dharmas. Each Foundation includes a variety of objects, meditations, and contemplations. When practicing āsana, we can choose to devote our practice to any one of these, or work through them sequentially.

First Foundation

Mindfulness of "the body within the body" is the First Foundation of Mindfulness. This phrasing reminds us that we are not distant observers of the body, with awareness located in our heads observing our body as an object, but rather awareness permeates the whole body, like a sponge saturated with water. This is a kind of samādhi since the sense of separation between subject and object is dissolved.

The Buddha's first instruction is to bring mindfulness to breathing. With no manipulation or controlling of it, we're encouraged to simply *know* an in-breath as an in-breath, an out-breath as an out-breath. We become intimately familiar with the experience of breathing, noticing the various and varying qualities such as deep or shallow, fast or slow, rough or smooth, even or uneven, long or short. As mindfulness is a friendly, nonjudgmental, fully accepting kind of attention, we are already cultivating a transcendence of the pairs of opposites.

Then, expanding our awareness to include the whole body including its posture, movement, and parts, we deepen our sense of embodiment. The body and breath do not get lost in the future or the past, so if attention is fully absorbed in the body, there is a fully integrated sense of presence. The body and breath keep us anchored to *now.* Only when we become entangled and identified with thinking can we feel distant from life. This is one import of Patañjali's opening sūtra: "Now, the teachings of Yoga."[9]

When practicing postures, we stay fully present through mindfulness of the breath. When noticing the mind leaning away from our experience of an āsana, we can remember to come back to the breath. In this way, the breath becomes the sūtra—the thread—upon which we weave our practice. We see for ourselves how the posture and movement of the body "conditions" the breath. The qualities of the breath are conditioned by whether we are in a forward bend, a back bend, or a twist. If we maintain a posture, over time we will see a change in the breath. We can also see how the breath conditions the body. While in a forward bend, notice how the in-breath affects your experience and how the out-breath results in a different experience. You may even notice a subtle (or not so subtle) affecting of the movement and posture. All this points to a core teaching of the Buddha: as all phenomena are conditioned, there is no real autonomous "thing" to speak of! We say "breath" or "posture" as if these were things separate from the flow of experience, but through this practice we see they are processes, caused and conditioned, selfless and constantly changing.

Bringing attention to the parts of the body, we become cognizant of any reactivity to the various parts—which parts do we like? which parts do we dislike? We may feel revulsion contemplating our ear wax, feces, or lymph and prefer to contemplate our hair or our eyes. Yet those same eyes dangling from their sockets might provoke revulsion and fear; that hair clogged in our shower drain may seem disgusting. This practice shows us that our reactivity is conditioned.

Contemplating the five great elements (earth, water, fire, air, and space), we bring attention to the solidity of the body; its composition of various elements such as carbon—the very same carbon that gives us coal and diamonds. The liquid element, manifesting as blood, interstitial fluid, and other bodily fluids, is not separate from the water flowing in our rivers and streams and that falls as rain. Our bodies generate heat, and the food we ingest is literally the solar energy captured in the vegetables and flesh of animals. The air we breathe sustains our life, and all experience arises and passes away in space. Through contemplating the elements of the body the yogi begins to understand that life is not isolated in her own body, that there is no "self" separate from the interbeing of all the elements. The first mindfulness training[10] of ahiṁsā, or nonharming, reminds us to protect the lives of people, animals, plants, and minerals. As our bodies and our life cannot exist without these minerals, we begin to see that the distinction between organic and inorganic is ultimately conceptual—there is no real separation. In protecting the elements from degradation we protect ourselves. Before we "throw away" our garbage, we can ask ourselves, "Where is *away*?"

The final practice of the First Foundation is contemplating the decomposition of the body, the existential truth that this body is of the nature to die. Looking deeply into the impermanent nature of the body, we are motivated not to take life for granted, not to lose our life in distraction and dispersion. For those ready for this practice, the effect of this meditation is liberating. This is understandable in light of all the effort we make, the tension and strain we create in attempting to deny the only thing we know for certain—that we will die!

Second Foundation

With the Second Foundation, "feelings within the feelings," we deepen our *intimacy* with experience by bringing mindfulness to feelings—again, not as a dissociated observer, but from within the feelings themselves. The word *vedanā,* from which we get the term "feelings," means "sensations." Terms used to convey the meaning of *vedanā* are "feeling tone" or "felt sense."

To see for yourself what is meant here, put aside this book, close your eyes, and just sit, with your hands resting on your lap, palms down. Settle yourself into the experience, noting how it *feels* to sit here—physically and energetically. You may note such *feelings* as "heavy," "grounded," "stable," "dull," or other feelings. Then, maintaining your attention, turn your palms upward and note if there's a change in the feeling tone. You may find yourself feeling "light," "open," "receptive," or "vulnerable," among other possible feelings.

Such feelings are not emotions. They are a bridge between the physical and the mental. Feelings are a primal experience, which the Buddha points out *precedes* any reaction or emotion. The importance of bringing mindfulness to feelings, or sensations, cannot be overestimated. It is at the junction between feeling and reactivity that mindfulness provides the possibility of freely choosing how to respond to any given situation.

Feelings are categorized as being pleasant, unpleasant, or neutral. They can be of a physiological or a psychological nature. If you bite into a ripe, juicy lemon, the sensations that arise are of a physiological nature; if you simply imagine doing so, the sensations that arise are of a psychological nature. It is interesting to realize that the body reacts to imagining biting into the lemon in a similar way to actually doing so. In all yogic teaching, thoughts are considered as important as, or even more important than, physical action. The psyche reacts to imagination as if the stimulus is "really" being experienced, and recent neuroscience shows the same areas of the brain activated whether you do some action or merely visualize yourself doing so.

The Buddha noted that feelings condition our whole world. We spend huge amounts of energy trying to create and prolong pleasant feelings while pushing away and trying to avoid unpleasant feelings, and we become confused, bored, or simply "checked out" when experiencing neutral feelings. This grasping, aversion, and ignorance, called the "three poisons," are the roots of duḥkha that taint the experience of life. If mindfulness is not present, feelings quickly give rise to moods, emotions, perceptions, ideas, and whole stories and identities that cause duḥkha for us and for those with whom we interact.

Hatha Yoga practice can either help us grow in awareness and insight or create duḥkha, depending on whether mindfulness is present or not. For example, when practicing an āsana we enjoy, experiencing the pleasure of a sensuous stretch or the psychological pleasure of the "successful" performance of a challenging posture, if we are not mindful, we will get caught in craving and clinging, seeking to prolong or repeat the feeling as soon as it wanes (as it most assuredly will, all phenomena being impermanent). Such clinging after the pleasant takes us out of the moment, creating a felt sense of separation, and may even lead to harm if we overstretch. While it is indeed a pleasure to accomplish a challenging posture, without mindfulness, as the *Gherandha-Samhitā* warns, āsana practice becomes an obstacle to liberation because the ego gratification is clung to, and identification with ego and the body becomes more rigid and solid. We get caught in pride and our identity as someone who can do "advanced postures." When conditions change (through illness, injury, or age) and we can no longer do what we used to do, we can become discouraged and even suffer despair.

Practicing challenging postures, we may experience unpleasant feelings. Mindfulness shows us how quickly the mind seeks to push the unpleasant away, to eliminate it. Such aversion creates tension that is often more painful than the original sensation. The Buddha referred to this added anguish as "the second arrow." The first arrow is the experience of discomfort or pain; the second arrow is the tension, anguish, and unease of our aversion.

Bringing awareness to neutral feelings cultivates greater clarity about our experience. In fact, most of our experience is neutral, neither pleasant nor unpleasant. Because this is so, we spend much of our time seeking intensity of feeling, or falling into boredom. Through greater awareness of the neutral aspect of experience, we avoid the common pitfall of "globalization" whereby we take an experience and make it larger than it is. We say things like "My back is killing me," when closer observation shows us that it's a small area of the lower right lumbar that is painful and the rest of the back is neutral. This insight alone relieves us of much added duḥkha.

Zen's understanding of "pure practice" is to not add anything extra to the experience. If we bring mindfulness to our feelings, we can experience "pure joy" or "pure pleasure," untainted by clinging or grasping. But in order to be able to experience pure pleasure, we must be willing to experience "pure pain" or "pure discomfort," free of aversion and resistance.

The most pain-avoidant people have the least joy in their lives. In trying to armor ourselves against pain, we numb ourselves to all experience. In opening ourselves to felt experience, we allow ourselves to live life fully, not caught in patterned habits of reactivity. Rather than conditionally reacting to experience, we can choose to respond creatively. The doorway to this freedom is in bringing mindfulness to our feelings *before* they condition our reactivity.

Third Foundation

The *Dhammapada*'s opening lines point to the importance of mind in creating the lived experience of our world:

> Our life is shaped by our mind;
> all actions are led by mind; created by mind.
> Duḥkha follows an unskillful thought
> as the wheels of a cart follow the oxen that draw it.
> Sukha follows a skillful thought
> as surely as one's shadow.[11]

The Buddha taught that actions are preceded by volitions that can create wholesome or unwholesome consequences. This is the teaching of karma; there are consequences to our actions. The Zen ceremony of atonement (at-onement) reminds us that we are ultimately the authors of our "fate." When we are at one with our actions, we can never think of ourselves as victims. Rather than blaming external conditions for duḥkha, we realize that the ultimate cause of duḥkha is found in the mind—the same place liberation is found.

In turning attention to the activity of the mind, all psychological phenomena, the contents and activities of mind, are included: emotions, perceptions, conceptualization, imagination, and discrimination—the citta-samskāra, or "mental formations." Citta or mind is the totality of these ever-changing psychological phenomena, not a thing or unchanging subject.

With mindfulness of the mental formations, the Buddha directs us to "know" when a mental formation is present and when it is not present. Mindfulness itself is a mental formation, so we can be aware when mindfulness is present, as well as when it is not. When not mindful of mental formations, we believe and identify with them. As soon as we recognize a mental formation as a mental formation, it loses much—or all—of its power over us. When mindfulness is there, the mental formation has already been transformed. No longer is there only anger, now there is also mindfulness of the anger. The situation is changed as soon as we are mindful of it, no longer lost in forgetfulness, no longer identified as anger.

While practicing āsana, mindfulness of the mental formations provides a wonderful opportunity to observe and recognize our mental patternings and how they condition our habitual tendencies. The body is not completely symmetrical. You may find one side in a posture easier than the other side. Noticing how quickly the mind categorizes experience into "good" and "bad" can free you from believing these potentially limiting notions. As an old Zen saying puts it, "With one thought, heaven and hell are created."

Pain or discomfort often arises during āsana practice. Much discomfort is really just a reaction to novelty, and much pain is the pain of change. Such pain can provide an opportunity to grow in mindfulness. Truly injurious or excessive pain should never be ignored, but the truth is, most of the pain that one experiences in āsana practice is merely discomfort and not injurious. With discomfort, it is fruitful to drop out of our aversive reactivity and bring a gently embracing quality of mindfulness to the discomfort. When we do this, we see for ourselves that there really is a difference between pain and suffering—the misery and mental anguish that we add to the experience because of our aversion. This is an important insight with real benefit to life off the mat.

You practice with the discomfort and pain that arises in āsana practice so that you can remain free from suffering throughout your life. Yes, if you feel discomfort in your shoulders while doing Warrior Two, all you need do to relieve the pain is lower your arms. But if you always do this, what will you do with the pain that you cannot avoid through such a simple strategy? What if you are injured in an accident? Or you lose your lover? Or you must face your own sickness, old age, and death? Whether emotional or physical, embodiment means pain is inevitable. Working with mindfulness of the mind means that when the inevitable losses of life occur, you can just *feel* the pain and not add suffering as well.

The Buddha encourages us to notice the mind when liberation or "letting go" is present. But first, we need to have clarity about what a grasping mind *feels* like. Yoga is not an ideology, philosophy, or moral code about the "goodness" of letting go and the "badness" of attachment. Letting go is what happens when the suffering of holding on is *felt* and recognized.

The most obvious attachment is to material objects and sensory pleasures, including possessions and sensual and sexual sensations. Attachment to particular "feel-good" experiences, such as the potentially seductive enjoyment of stretching and moving the body or the excitement of accomplishment, are some examples, as is the "Yoga buzz" many practitioners seek in their practice. There's nothing wrong with enjoying physical pleasure, but if we are dominated by our attachment to pleasure, we *will* suffer when it dissipates.

Another type of attachment is to opinions, beliefs, views, and theories. While practicing āsana, we may find ourselves attached to ideas about what we "should" be able to do, what we "should" be feeling, and the correct form of the āsana. We may find ourselves caught in a belief about what we cannot do or what we will "never be able to do." Again, ideas and opinions are not the issue; it's the degree of our attachment to them that creates suffering. If we are attached to strong ideas about what we need in order to be happy and free, the attachment to those very ideas becomes an obstacle to happiness and freedom. We place ourselves in bondage to our ideas and concepts, missing the possibility for happiness and freedom here and now.

There can be attachment to practice itself! The Buddha strongly warned against getting attached to ritual and traditional practices—secular *or* religious. It is possible to become so attached to a particular form of practice that you remain in your comfort zone, never testing your edges. The form becomes a trap rather than a tool for liberation. To appreciate and be firm in one's commitment to a particular practice is one thing, but if you become overly attached and obsessive with the form, you can all too easily lose the liberating spirit of the practice.

The most challenging attachment includes everything that we can identify as "I," "me," or "mine." Even becoming attached to our identity as a yogi can become a source of duḥkha. We can develop a holier-than-thou attitude, seeing ourselves as separate and above others.

Mindfulness shows how one creates a sense of self through reactivity, belief patterns, and dramatizing story lines. It happens in the instant a student marks out "her" spot in the practice room with her mat. The more attached we are to our stories of self, the more tension and suffering we create, but it's not until we really see this for ourselves that any opening can occur.

Fourth Foundation

The Fourth Foundation, mindfulness of the dharmas, provides the context of bringing mindfulness to specific mental qualities, and analyzing experience into categories that constitute core aspects of the Buddha's Dharma (or teaching). These classifications are not in themselves the objects of meditation, but are frameworks or points of reference to be applied during contemplation to whatever experiences arise while practicing.

The dharmas listed in the *Satipaṭṭhāna Sutta* are the five hindrances, the five aggregates, the six sense spheres, the seven factors of awakening, and the Four Noble Truths. While one can contemplate these dharmas while practicing āsanas, I find that for most practitioners, it's too easy to fall into abstraction or intellectualization unless they already have a mature mindfulness practice.

More accessible is following the teaching of the *Ānāpānasati Sutta,* where contemplation of the dharmas takes the form of bringing mindfulness to the impermanent nature of all phenomena. Contemplation of impermanence is a dharma gate opening to the understanding of the interdependent, conditioned, and selfless nature of all that exists.

Āsana practice offers a great window into impermanence. From day to day, the body feels and moves differently each time we come to practice. We know things change, yet we put so much effort and energy into trying to live life as if that were not so! This is avidyā, "not seeing" as a kind of denial. But ignoring or denying the truth of impermanence perpetuates suffering and misery, whereas opening to the reality of change liberates that energy.

We look into the impermanent nature of all the earlier objects of meditation, starting with the breath. No two breaths are the same. Even within one inhalation, there is constant movement and change. There is no "thing" that is actually the breath that can be grasped and held on to. Every sensation we experience, no matter whether pleasant, unpleasant, or neutral is impermanent, as is every emotion, thought, or perception.

Changeless life is a sterile concept, yet without mindfulness so many of us live as if such a life were possible!

In *Genjo Koan* Zen Master Dōgen writes, "If you examine myriad things with a confused body-mind, you might suppose that your mind and nature are permanent. When you practice intimately and return to where you are, it will be clear that nothing at all has unchanging self."[12] If "self" is understood as an entity that is autonomous, independent, and persistent over time, then insight into impermanence leads inevitably to the clear view that all things lack such an unchanging self. Even the consciousness of self that we take such pains to protect and bolster is not an autonomous, independent, persistent thing or entity; it is a process that is in constant flux, conditioned by everything else that is in constant change. This insight into "nonself" (anatta) is what is meant by the term *emptiness* (śūnyatā). Emptiness means that we, and all phenomena, are empty of a separately existing, enduring self.

Because we are empty of a separate self, we inter-are with everything else. This is the Buddha's unique contribution to the Yoga tradition: dependent co-origination. As you read these words on the page, can you see the tree from which the paper comes? The tree's ancestors? The earth, the nutriments, the rain, the sun? For this page of paper to exist, all those conditions and more are needed, including the loggers, the paper-mill processors, the truckers, the printers, the publisher. And consciousness, "mine" and "yours," are all here *now.*

The Buddha said that when we enter through the door of impermanence, we touch nirvāṇa, here and now. Nirvāṇa, meaning "extinction," is the extinction of our notions and ideas about reality and how it should or shouldn't be, so that we may perceive reality as it is. Our grasping and aversion, our greed, anger, and delusion are extinguished. Also extinguished are our attachment and bondage to concepts such as birth and death, existent and nonexistent, increasing and decreasing, pure and impure.

Through penetrating the reality of impermanence, our grasping after ephemeral phenomena weakens. A taste of this can happen in the time it takes to work with one āsana. Maintaining Warrior Two, unpleasant sensations may arise in our shoulders. These sensations lead to aversion, and grasping after relief. We identify with the unpleasant sensations and think, "My shoulders are killing me." Thoughts arise about the teacher having us hold the posture "too long," never seeing that "too long" is a relative concept. Clinging to that belief creates a sense of self; the more we cling, the more the self suffers.

Shifting our attention to the impermanent nature of experience, we see that there is no-thing personal about any of it. There is just sensation, and the sensation is ever-changing. It is all a dependently co-originated process, and through practice we see that the same is true for all feelings, mental formations, and consciousness.

With this insight comes nirodha (cessation). This is the Third Noble Truth of the Buddha, often used as a synonym for nirvāṇa and also Patañjali's definition of Yoga. Practicing āsana, we may notice many small cessations. We may experience a pleasant sensation and the arising of a mental formation. With mindfulness, we see attachment, and based upon an awareness of impermanence, the attachment fades away. It happens once, and then again and again. Over time, the fading away continues until that particular attachment ceases. This is a small, but potentially profound, taste of liberation.

Finally comes *letting go.* But there is also the insight that it is not *you* who lets go. Throughout practice, there was still that final vestige of self-consciousness that could take credit for the insight into impermanence, and cessation. The final thing to let go of is the idea of a separate enduring self. The irony is that this is a letting go of what was never there!

Letting go does not mean letting go of one thing in order to grasp something else. Letting go means to see through all that keeps us (falsely) separated from reality as it is. The supposed boundary between us and ultimate reality, between "self" and "other," is seen as not real. Nothing needs to be removed or added or joined together! Enlightenment and liberation come not in turning away from our human condition, but within it, *and* as its fulfillment. This letting go of enlightenment is to be with whatever is happening, free of personal agenda. When the desire arises that something be other than it is, we see through it to its fading away and ceasing.

> To practice the Buddha way is to investigate the self. To investigate the self is to forget the self. To forget the self is to be intimate with the myriad things. When intimate with the myriad things, your bodymind as well as the body-minds of others drops away. No trace of realization remains, and this no-trace continues endlessly.
>
> —Dōgen Zenji, *Genjo Koan*[12]

12

THE BODY OF TRUTH

AJAHN AMARO BHIKKHU

PALI SCRIPTURE ABBREVIATIONS:

D = *Digha Nikāya* (Long Discourses of the Buddha)

M = *Majjhima Nikāya* (Middle-Length Discourses of the Buddha)

S = *Samyutta Nikāya* (Discourses of the Buddha Collected by Subject)

Dhp = *Dhammapada* (a poetic collection of core teachings of the Buddha)

A striking aspect of Buddhist philosophy, when first encountered by the Western mind, is that in the four standard patterns the Buddha used to describe the fabric of the human condition within the natural order of things, the mental and physical dimensions are not distinguished from each other in any radical sense. Their roles in an integrated spectrum of qualities are assumed and pass without discussion.

Dimensions of Nature

The first of these patterns is the simplest of all the four expressions—nāmarūpa—variously translated as "materiality/mentality" or "mind-and-body." It is a single word that is copiously used in the texts of the Southern Buddhist tradition (the Buddhism of Thailand, Sri Lanka, Burma, Laos, and Cambodia, recorded in the Pali language, a close relative of Sanskrit) to refer to the mind-body complex, the material and nonmaterial aspects of all living beings.

The second of these standard formats, one that teases out the qualities of nāmarūpa in more detail, is most commonly known as the five aggregates. This might come across as an odd term, being a translation of the Pali term *khandha*, but it is one that has no convenient and all-purpose rendering in English. The word *aggregate* essentially means "a group," or "a heap," but its very indistinctness seems to have been chosen by the Buddha for very practical purposes.

It is used to express the idea that the mental and material complex that we call "a person" can be roughly chunked into this spectrum of five interrelated categories. These five are as follows: (1) the body or physical form (rūpa); (2) feeling or physical sensation (vedanā); (3) perception (saññā); (4) mental formations, including thoughts, emotions, and intentions (saṅkhāra); and lastly (5) consciousness, the faculty of cognition itself (viññana).

These are all seen as intrinsically interrelated since everything that is experienced and known about the body is apprehended via the agency of the mind, through feeling, perception, and consciousness; similarly (at least in this world!), without the physical basis of the body, the four mental factors of the nāma-khandhas have no vehicle and life source. The scriptural teachings further state:

> Feeling, perception and consciousness are conjoined, not disjoined, and it is impossible to separate each of these from the others in order to specify the differences between them.[1]

The third of the patterns that the Buddha
most frequently of all in his teachings, is that known
in Pali the āyatana. These consist, predictably, of t
refer to in the West—eye, ear, nose, tongue, and bo
that of "mind" (mano). Again, this inclusion is tota
and no qualification is felt to be needed. It is seen
cession of attributes: the eye perceives light, the ear sound, the nose odors, the tongue flavors, the body sensations, the mind mental objects (dhamma). This latter quality refers to the entire array of mental events, including thoughts, memories, dreams, emotions, decisions, and so on.

The one unique attribute that the mind-sense (man-āyatana) is ascribed, in the Buddhist scheme of things, is that unlike the other senses, which receive their stimulation from without (for example, light comes from an external object that is detected by the eye), the mind-sense is both the producer and the perceiver of its objects. It is both the thought creator and the thought knower. It is further seen to function as the coordinator of the six senses—it draws all the threads together and weaves a coherent picture of the world from these—a role that, interestingly, is largely corroborated by the findings of modern neuroscience.

The last of the principal formats that the Buddha employed to portray the human condition is known as the elements—in Pali, the dhātu. The term is most regularly confined to the four attributes of the material world: earth (pathavī), water (āpo), fire (tejo), and wind (vāyo)—these embodying, respectively, the qualities of solidity; cohesion; temperature and the life force; and lastly, vibration. However, in a number of significant teachings (for example in "The Exposition on the Elements," M 140), the term *dhātu* is used to refer to the whole mind-body complex, and the elements are increased in number to six, for along with the standard first four, the Buddha includes the space element (ākāsa-dhātu), and the consciousness element (viññāna-dhātu).

In a sense these four patterns can be seen simply as different ways of slicing the pie of the natural order: To call it all "materiality/mentality" des the pie in two, with the material qualities on one side and the nonmaterial on the other. The "five aggregates" structure slices this same nonmaterial side into four rough chunks, leaving the material side as is. The "six senses" arrangement gives us five different pieces on the material side and one extra-rich one on the nonmaterial side. Lastly, the "six elements" approach gives us the same number of slices but cut in a form similar to the "five aggregates"—this time, however, the material qualities get subdivided into four, with "consciousness" serving to encompass the entire mental realm but with the "space element" being argued over as to which class it properly falls into. That last piece of pie can often be a cause of dissent.

In reflecting on these varying configurations, it should be clear that within the Buddhist view of things the idea of there being a substantial division between body and mind is an absurdity. Yes, red and blue can viably be called different colors, but the most significant value they possess is that they are both parts of a natural array of characteristics. They are simply dimensions of an underlying natural order.

Mindfulness of the Body

The deeply interrelated and interpenetrating relationship between the physical and mental aspects of our being was seen as so significant to the Buddha that he repeatedly underscored it, and developed meditation practices around it, to assist his students in fully realizing their spiritual potential. This emphasis was most regularly phrased as "mindfulness of the body." A couple of quotations from the Pali scriptures illustrate this clearly:

> Anyone who has developed and cultivated mindfulness of the body has included within themselves whatever wholesome states there are that play a part in true knowledge. Just as anyone who has extended their mind over the great ocean has included within that whatever streams there are that flow into the ocean.[2]

> What, monks, is the path leading to the Unconditioned [the realization of enlightenment]? Mindfulness directed to the body: this is called the path leading to the Unconditioned.[3]

This latter passage is the very first in a collection of forty-four discourses by the Buddha on the Unconditioned and the pathway to it, which indicates the centrality and importance that he gave to this kind of practice.

In a similar vein, in "The Discourse on the Foundations of Mindfulness," which is universally regarded as the cornerstone of meditation within the Southern School of Buddhism (otherwise known as the Theravāda tradition, meaning "The Way of the Elders"), the practice of mindfulness of the body is given an identical, opening role:

> Monks, this is the direct path for the purification of beings, for the overcoming of sorrow and distress, for the dissolution of pain and grief, for the reaching of the true way, for the realization of nirvāṇa—namely, the Four Foundations of Mindfulness.
>
> What are the four? Here one abides contemplating the body as a body, ardent, fully aware, and mindful, having put aside hankering and fretting about the world . . . feelings as feelings . . . mind as mind . . . mind objects as mind objects . . . ."[4]

From here, in this discourse, the Buddha goes on to give further details about the various aspects of mindfulness of the body for the largest part of his explanation. These aspects include such essential meditation practices as mindfulness of breathing, particularly as a concentration exercise, but they also cover what are generally considered ordinary attributes of everyday life.

Who would consider the simple noting of the posture that the body is in to be a significant spiritual practice? Yet the Buddha recommended this very explicitly, to be aware "I am walking" or "I am standing," "I'm sitting" or "I'm lying down"—just this can be enough to key the attention into the reality of the present moment and to help attune one to the state of both body and mind. Then, through that attunement, an integration or harmonization can more easily occur.

Another of these everyday practices that this teaching recommends is "acting in full awareness"—this is termed sati-sampajañña in Pali. This means being fully attentive to ordinary activities such as going somewhere and returning; looking ahead and looking away; dressing and undressing; eating, drinking, tasting; using the bathroom; falling asleep and waking up; talking and keeping silent . . . in short, throughout the absolutely unexceptional flow of our days.

Again, on paper, this might look oddly unremarkable as a spiritual discipline, nevertheless it is encouraged with the same heartful vigor as the Buddha gives to the development of profound states of meditation and liberating insights.

So, there is the question: Why should such a weight of significance be given to these aspects of our world? Isn't enlightenment, in the Buddhist view, about an exalted, transcendent state of mind? If so, why bother paying so much attention to the body?

If we labor under the view that enlightenment, or liberation, is solely a mental event, not involving the material dimension of the natural order, then we find sooner or later that the material realm seems to be doing its very best to intrude upon our would-be transcendent state. That damned howling dog across the valley that keeps ruining my concentration! That bad knee that won't let me sit in meditation for more than twenty minutes without screaming for relief . . .

What about the kind of withdrawal of the senses advocated in certain Vedic and Buddhist practices—where the mind disengages completely from the sense realm—isn't this to be a regarded as a state of liberation?

These kinds of states can certainly be realized, through intense application and effort; however, it is very noticeable, at least within the Buddhist tradition, that such states are always underlined as being wholesome but temporary. The central position, in terms of spiritual training and the development of the attributes that genuinely liberate, goes over and over again to our earthy, mundane friend "mindfulness of the body."

The Present—Full of Useful Possibilities

It is a common tendency for us as human beings—as long as our physical safety is not being threatened—to drift off into our favored mental realms of fantasy, nostalgia, regret, resentment, anxiety, or future planning. If we happen to be an adept meditator, we might also add to that list deep states of concentration and blissful, radiant zones of consciousness.

It was because of this pronounced tendency that the Buddha saw it as being crucial to a genuine understanding of the way life works, and for the development of a spiritual path that could lead to an ultimate quality of well-being, that we awaken to the interrelated nature of mind and body. In other words, he saw that an enlightenment that tried to ignore the physical dimension could never be a real enlightenment.

He thus encouraged the kinds of practices that would keep the body in view at all times, that would keep the mind full of the body. This effort serves a couple of related functions: firstly, it helps sustain a continuity of one's spiritual efforts. This is very useful since one can recognize early on that the more mindful we are, the less we tend to make problems about the way things are. Sadly the reverse is true too; the more heedless we are, the more complicated and struggle-filled we make life for ourselves. Thus the more unbroken the quality of mindfulness is, the more we are able to live harmoniously.

Secondly, the body only exists in the present moment; it doesn't wander off into the past and future. This might seem like an insignificant truism; however, when we start to look at our lives closely, we find that much of our difficulty and distress arises from dwelling on re-creations of the past—either positive or negative—or on hopes and worries about the future.

Despite the fact that, to the thinking mind, the past and future seem like vast and solid realities, stretching out evenly before and after this insignificant little present, the closer we look at the experience of our life as it actually is, the more we see the past and future as hollow fabrications. They are mere memories and anticipations, and it is rather the present that is vast and all-encompassing, and full of useful possibilities. How strange . . . did something change here, or has it always been this way and we had just not noticed it to be so?

Either way, since the body is always in the present, the simple recollection of its presence is a surefire method to key the attention into the reality of the way things actually are. If we are off trying to inhabit an imagined future or a reconstituted past, how can we possibly attune to the orchestra of life in the here-and-now? Our common sense tells us it can't be done. What is more, when we use the body to help us to wake up to the present, there is a completely natural quality of easeful delight that we experience—just like coming out of the realm of sleep in the early morning—"Oh, that was only a dream, now I'm back to reality."

Life in the Forest

The style of Buddhist practice that I have been a part of for the last thirty years is generally known as the Thai Forest Tradition.

In a way the forest meditation tradition predates even the Buddha. Before his time, in India and the Himalayan region, it was not uncommon for those who sought spiritual liberation to leave the life of the town and village and resort to the mountains and forest wildernesses. As a gesture of leaving worldly values behind, it made perfect sense: the forest was a wild, natural place and the only people who were to be found there were the criminal, the insane, the outcast, and the renunciant religious seekers—it was a sphere outside the influence of materialistic cultural norms and thus ideal for the cultivation of the aspects of the spirit that transcended them.

When the Bodhisattva left the life of the palace at the age of twenty-nine, it was to move into the forest and to train in the yogic disciplines that were available in his time. The story is well known how he became dissatisfied with the teachings of his first instructors and left them to find his own way. He did so, discovering that primal chord of Truth he named the Middle Way under the shade of the bodhi tree, beside the River Nerañjara, at what is now Bodh Gaya, in Bihar State, India.

It is frequently stated that the Buddha was born in a forest, was enlightened in a forest, lived and taught his whole life in a forest, and finally passed away in a forest. When choice was possible, it was the environment he opted to live in since, as he would say, "Tathāgatas delight in secluded places."[5] The lineage now known as the Thai Forest Tradition tries to live in the spirit of the way espoused by the Buddha himself, and to practice according to the same standards he encouraged during his lifetime. It is a branch of the Southern School of Buddhism.

Along with a number of hours in the day being dedicated to the more familiar disciplines of formal meditation, such as mindfulness of breathing, and the development of wisdom through insight meditation (Vipassanā), the style of spiritual training in the Forest Tradition encompasses many of the approaches to cultivating mindfulness of the body that have already been outlined. Almost all who live within this form, or who have been associated with its teachings, would say that it is the linchpin of their practice.

My own teacher, Ajahn Chah, made strenuous efforts over the thirty-year period that he was actively guiding others, to stress the importance sustaining a continuity of mindfulness and of paying heedful attention to even the most mundane practicalities of everyday living. When I encountered him for the first time, in early 1978, he was, with cement trowel in hand, in the process of building a monastery toilet. It was clear at first sight that the finishing work was being executed to a meticulous standard of smoothness and that Ajahn was keenly opposed to things being done in a slapdash or haphazard way.

Over the years he repeatedly encouraged the development of this quality of mindfulness and full awareness, whether it be through sitting meditation, construction work, the morning walk through the villages to receive alms, the process of giving teachings, or the cleaning and maintenance of the monastery buildings; in fact, he often said that you could tell how accomplished the teacher at a monastery was by how well, or badly, the community looked after the bathrooms there.

Walking Meditation

Among the various aspects of spiritual training in the Forest Tradition, and particularly considering those that emphasize the physical dimension, there are two that particularly stand out—the first because it is not that well known as a meditation training outside of certain Buddhist circles, the second because it is often seen as an unnecessary corollary to the spiritual path.

For most people the word *meditation* immediately brings to mind an image of someone seated in the lotus posture with eyes gently closed, back erect, and countenance serene. Even when the most materialistic of corporations, such as car manufacturers, credit card companies, or life insurance brokers, want to convey a spiritual element to their promises, this is the archetypal image they use.

In many systems of Buddhist meditation, and particularly in the Forest Tradition, however, it is customary and considered highly beneficial to intersperse the periods of sitting meditation (usually for about an hour) with corresponding periods of walking meditation of an equal duration. This was a practice that the Buddha developed and sustained throughout his life.

The methodology is very simple:

You establish a path on as flat a piece of ground as you can find—ideally about twenty to twenty-five yards long—and determine what your two end points will be, say between a certain rock at one end and a large tree at the other. Before beginning the walking practice you stand still at one end of the path and sweep the attention up and down through your body, to establish an awareness of the body's presence and to relax before beginning. When a mindful awareness of the body has been made firm, you start walking.

There are a variety of different objects of reference that can be used for walking meditation—just as with sitting meditation—but generally the most accessible is simply the feeling of the feet touching the ground as one walks along at an easy, natural pace. As the mind wanders into memories and plans, or is distracted by the varying sights and sounds, you just keep letting go and returning the attention to the present moment, returning to the rhythm of the feet along the path.

In this way the body and its motions, oscillating between the two ends of the path, becomes like the feeling of the breath, oscillating between the inhalation and the exhalation. This natural cycle thus serves as a focal point, bringing the attention to the reality of the present, and is a calming influence for the many kinds of distracted thought.

When walking meditation is well developed, there can be found within it a stillness of being, a spiritual restfulness that is easily equivalent to that found in the more stationary sitting meditation. You find that there is a clear awareness of the movements of the body, but since awareness is always "here," there is a motionlessness that forms the environment of the motion. This is what Ajahn Chah would call being like "still, flowing water."[6]

Śīla as a Basis of Practice

The other aspect of the forest monastic life that bears a little highlighting, and that might not come to mind as a physical discipline, but which I would suggest most assuredly is, is that of personal conduct, or śīla in Pali.

Buddhist monastic life, even though it has the single aim of spiritual freedom, is very far from a "free and easy" one, at least in the way that the words are usually used. We have a lot of rules!

The multitude of rules have a single purpose, though, and this is to help keep life as simple as we know, in our heart of hearts, it can be. We have rules for every aspect of life, whether it is not to kill any animals, not to engage in sexual activity of any kind, or that we should repair a hole in our robe before dawn of the next day if it is big enough for a bedbug to crawl through.

If you add up all the rules in the book for fully ordained monastics, it comes to something like a total of ten thousand. This might sound unnecessarily daunting(!) but the fact of the matter is that once you get familiar with the style of life, most of the rules just keep themselves and the process of living by them does indeed make life extraordinarily straightforward: no more worries about what to do with your hair or what to wear today.

Their main role, then, becomes to help keep us mindful of the numerous potential digressions and sublimated urges—when we want to bend the truth for the sake of a good story, when we want to help ourselves to the contents of the refrigerator because of a flash of restless hunger—the presence of distinct guidelines helps us to see those impulses before they become behaviors.

Fortunately the Buddha was a great pragmatist and only set out such a detailed pattern of training for those who wished to commit themselves to a monastic style of life. For the vast majority of his students in his own lifetime, and similarly today, he recommended the standard of what is known as the five precepts. These are as follows:

1. I undertake the precept to refrain from taking the life of any living creature.
2. I undertake the precept to refrain from taking that which is not given.
3. I undertake the precept to refrain from sexual misconduct.
4. I undertake the precept to refrain from false and harmful speech.
5. I undertake the precept to refrain from intoxicating drink and drugs that lead to carelessness.[7]

When visitors go to monasteries in Theravāda countries, it is customary for them to recommit to these precepts as a simple and regular reminder. In the West, they are taken at the beginning and ending of retreats, at day-long sittings, and even before saṅgha meetings.

In a certain sense these five precepts were not just conjured up by the Buddha. They are part of the natural order. They aren't imposed as a Buddhist idea, nor are they unique to the Buddhist tradition.

Every country in the world has laws that enable human beings to function freely and harmoniously. These laws relate to respect for human life, to property, to the appropriate use of sexuality, and to honesty. The Buddha pointed out that they are innate to the human condition. If we take life, if we misappropriate things, if we take advantage of others—through our sexuality or by living indulgently—if we are deceitful or aggressive, harmful with our speech, then pain will intrinsically follow. In the opening verses of the *Dhammapada* it says,

> If you speak or act with a corrupt mind, then pain will follow, like the wheels of the cart following the ox that pulls it.[8]

The Buddha referred to these precepts as pakati-sīla—natural or genuine virtue. They are contrasted with pannatti-sīla—prescribed ethics; these are the product of local customs and religions or rules peculiar to certain professions, like the vast majority of the monastic rules described earlier.

I like to compare the five precepts to road signs, such as Dangerous Curve or Do Not Enter—Wrong Way or Slow. They are road signs for our life as human beings. They help us look and see that "Life is really this way, not that way."

These signs protect us from danger. They warn us where the obstacles are and help the heart stay on track. If we don't follow the road signs, we tend to get lost, problems start to multiply, and there is usually a lot of tension and frustration involved. But when we pay attention and follow the laws and road signs, there's flexibility, sensitivity to time and place, and we usually get where we're going.

The precepts should be understood in exactly the same way. We pick them up and use them as helpful guides through the areas of life where we lose our way most easily, where there is the most emotional charge: around issues of life and death, around property and ownership, around sexuality, around honesty and deceit, around speech and communication.

As with monastic training, the five precepts are not about morality alone, they are also a great mindfulness tool. We don't get a signal when we start to drift from clear awareness to heedlessness, do we? It's not as though we have a little warning light on the dashboard for when an aversion or some deluded state comes into existence. It is not like when we create a document on a computer, and the machine prints the file name and path, the date it was created and so forth. "This is a greed condition, third degree, generated at 15:41, 1-6-08." "This is a self-based deluded condition. . . ." They are not tagged like that.

But when we employ such tools as these five precepts, they let us know, they give a warning. As the heart drifts unwittingly into unawareness, deluded attractions, and negativities, there's a warning buzz in the system. It enables the heart to wake up before we lose sight of our innate purity, before the negative states have been compounded, and before we create major disharmonies.

To go back to the driving analogy, they are like the serrated strip at the side of the freeway that makes the wheels vibrate when we drift too far toward the hard shoulder: "Oops! Dozed off for a moment there. How did that happen? Better brighten up or I'll be in trouble and never make it."

This set of guidelines for our behavior has to do with the discipline of action and the way we work, the way our body and mind interacts with the material world and other beings. It is also about how to be happy, and through employing these guidelines we can see for ourselves how that happiness is a result of attuning our conduct to respect the lives and nature of others.

The Body of the Forest Teaches Us

A final aspect of forest monastic life to mention is, not surprisingly, that of the forest itself. There is a profound physicality involved in living in a wild environment (especially when, as at Abhayagiri Monastery, where I live, it's a half-mile walk and a five-hundred-foot climb between the meditation hall and my cabin). Furthermore, when we are surrounded by landscape that has not been crafted by human hand, when we are not caused to refer incessantly to our name or social role among other humans, when we can be just another creature in the forest, it changes our perspective on things.

The forest itself is recognized as our body, even the great earth itself. Its cycle of seasons, its moods of weather, reflect our own moods back to us, and all that we habitually think that we are—this body and mind separated from the world—is revealed as simply dynamic patterns of nature, irrespective of whether they are conventionally called "inside" or "outside," "me" or "the world."

The very changeability and uncertain nature of forest life—when will those foxes come to visit again?—becomes the most profound of wisdom teachings. When the heart relaxes and opens to such uncertainty, it is recognized that the search for predictability in the naturally unpredictable can only produce disappointment.

When, instead, we let go, recognizing that that uncertainty is part of the intrinsic nature of all things, mysteriously we find a quality of attunement in our entire being. Body and mind resonate that primal harmonious chord that the Buddha called the Middle Way. We realize that everything that we are is an attribute of nature, of ultimate truth itself. How, we wonder, could it not be?

This sounds great on paper, but it is by no means easy to feel this way all the time, or even occasionally—why so?

The Body of Truth and the Body of Fear

One of the aspects of all our lives that causes discord is our routine identification with emotional states. Given a little practice with concentration exercises and before long most people can recognize that a passing thought is just like that car passing along the street, or that howling dog across the valley. At first it's just once in a while, but soon we can see and let those go as being insubstantial on a fairly consistent basis.

If the thought is emotionally loaded, just as if the sound of the car or the dog is—"They're not supposed to drive up here when the meditation is going on, I forgot to put out the sign. Everyone is going to hate me!" or "That damned dog; they promised to keep it quiet!"—then it's a very different story.

Our society reveres clear thinking, but emotionally most of us are very muddy. We easily get lost in feelings of resentment or guilt, excitement or anxiety, depression or elation, and so forth. In addition, we tend to relate to these states as being what we are rather than something that we're experiencing: "I am happy," "I am lonely," "I am distraught!" "I am afraid," rather than "I feel happy/lonely/distraught/afraid," or, even more realistically, "There is the feeling of happiness/loneliness/distress/fear."

Thus in meditation, for many people, it may be reasonably easy to put random chattering thoughts aside, but if they are emotionally charged, we rapidly get lost in the story. The ten thousand tales of what I should have done, what she might do, what he did to hurt me, what I should have said to her, and so on ad infinitum—before we know it we're tangled in a suffocating web of self-created imaginings.

There are a great variety of practices that contribute to mindfulness of the body. One of the most valuable of these might be most accurately referred to as "feeling and knowing the mind in the body" or "embodying the mind." We can use this practice as one way to help us establish much greater clarity in this area of our lives, not through any kind of suppression or distraction but rather through the realm of feeling and a mindful, radical acceptance.

This meditation is usually first developed as a practice in the sitting posture, but later, when it is more deeply established, it can be applied in all situations. To begin with it requires that there be a certain level of mental tranquillity, so, unfortunately, this is not a method for total beginners to meditation. Having said that, once it is possible for a person to establish an average degree of calm, to keep the mind reasonably focused in the present moment, it can be used quite effectively.

Embodying the Mind— The Case of Fear

Say for example that you feel you have a particular problem with fear, that your basic relationship with life is, "If it exists, worry about it!"

Your habit is to think in terms of "I have got a fear problem. I am a very anxious person. How can I get rid of my fear? If I could get rid of it, then there would be me without the fear and then I would be happy." It all sounds reasonable enough. . . . So you wish to investigate this quality of fear and to understand it.

When you next have some time to sit and meditate, you begin by simply relaxing the body as much as possible around the spine, which is upright but not tense. Take the first ten minutes or so to sweep the attention up and down through the body, relaxing it completely, then focusing finally upon the natural rhythm of the breath.

Let the whole system settle as much as possible in order to establish the qualities of calm and clarity. When you feel that there is a full sense of tranquillity and the mind is undistracted from the present, deliberately bring into consciousness a memory of either a frightening event, the thought or image of a person who customarily intimidates you, or the prospect of a future event that is worrying; the stronger the better.

As soon as you have triggered the fear reaction by recalling that face, that terrible event, very consciously let go of all the verbiage, the conceptual thought that wants to take hold of the story and run. This takes some considerable resolution, but it's a crucial piece of the practice.

Our habit is to leap immediately into the stories we tell ourselves and not notice what we're actually feeling. We thus need to let go very deliberately of the words and to seek in the body where we feel the feeling of fear itself.

Is it in your jaw, with your teeth clenched tight? Is it in your shoulders, hunched up around your ears? Is it in your belly, the solar plexus knotted into a dense wad? Where is it? How does it feel? Is it hot? Is it shaking? Is it dead and cold? Can you tell?

Different people have different emotional maps written in their bodies, so every one of us will have our own variation. There are a few general patterns, though, and, in this example, fear is most often felt as tightness in the abdomen, a knotting of the diaphragm and the solar plexus area.

If this is where you feel the sensation of fear, then bring your attention to settle at that spot. If you hear the mind starting up with thoughts such as "I have got a fear problem. I've got to get rid of this!" gently but firmly say to yourself, "No, right now there's simply this feeling of fear—it's a presumption to call it 'my problem.'"

To the best of your ability, keep the attention just on the physical sensation within the belly and do not to let the mind verbalize around that. Explore it and be interested in it. What you will soon find, and probably be surprised at, is that the feeling is not that uncomfortable. It's certainly not pleasant, it's not supposed to be, but it is far less irksome or painful than, say, a toothache, let alone a migraine.

Witness and allow yourself to fully know that sensation in the belly, open the heart to it, and accept it as it is. Recognize that it is simply one of the many feelings that can be experienced within this body and mind. It is part of the natural order. It is very important to recognize that you are not trying to make yourself like this feeling, or to call it good. In fact it's best to refrain from all judgments around it if possible, other than "Here it is"—no story. You are simply feeling the body of fear, the fear-filled body. The more radically, simply, and mindfully you can accept this sensation in your belly, the more completely the process will help to clarify things for you.

Once there is a clear and mindful openness to the raw sensation of the fear, consciously let yourself know this and stay with that knowing for a substantial period of time, at least five or ten minutes if possible. If the chosen catalyst was a potent one, whereas it might only take ten seconds to trigger the reaction, after it has been sustained consciously like this for a few minutes it might take another thirty minutes to let the system wind down, but this is what you need to do next. It should not be pushed.

With the ending of that conscious holding period, set the intention to relax the belly and to release all vestiges of the memory or mental image that was used to launch the process. The breath can be used very helpfully here, with a particular focusing on the exhalation being employed to support the letting-go, relinquishing attribute of the progression. Be very careful that you don't get into a rush, even surreptitiously, to get rid of the feeling. Let it fade in its own time.

If there is any reflexive tightening of the solar plexus area again, keep softening it and using the natural flow of the breath to sustain the dissolution of the effects of the fear reaction.

Stay patiently with this decompression and relaxation part of the cycle until you realize that the system is back at the state of clarity and calm that you began with. Once you are "back there," at ease, at the still point of the present, stay with this for a few minutes before ending the meditation. Or, of course, if you feel another round would be valuable and your knees can cope with it, you can drop another seed-crystal into the mind and launch the whole process again—and follow it through accordingly.

Not only does the development of this process have a beneficial effect on us mentally, according to current research it also changes the neurological pathways—we are literally rewiring our whole being, both physical and mental.

Responsiveness rather than Reactivity

There is a passage in one of the *Upaniṣads* that aptly illustrates this relationship between ego-centeredness and fear; Joseph Campbell summarizes it thus:

> In the beginning . . . there was only the Self; but it said "I" (Sanskrit *aham*) and immediately felt fear, after which, desire.[9]

In the pattern of experience that is being witnessed here, we are watching the fear feeling being born from the empty mind, bursting into being, and evolving; in its characteristics it is one embodiment of the isolated self-feeling. It is then seen, felt, and known as having come from nothing, doing its piece, and then dissolving back into nothing once again. Moreover, all along the way, the whole cycle was known and accepted as simply nature in action, the truth of the way things are. It is thus seen and known as an embodiment of truth.

The key transforming element in this entire process is the heartful, mindful quality of acceptance. In that open-hearted acceptance and knowing there is a profound, nonconceptual recognition that that fear feeling is "all right," in the most literal sense of the words—it's all part of the same natural order—and that there is indeed no thing to be afraid of.

The fear is part of nature; it's uncomfortable when it's present, for sure, but it is fundamentally not a problem—how could it be?

Another aspect of the transforming quality of this kind of practice is that once we have wholeheartedly accepted the simple, monosyllabic message of the feeling, we have to some extent also accepted where it came from. Having drunk from the stream, we have drunk from the source of the stream also.

This is to say, we have accepted and attuned ourselves, in some small way, to a quality that we were previously blind to and out of harmony with—the thing that caused the imbalance in the first place. Unconscious, fearful attitudes, for example, produce stressful self-preservation reactions. To have attuned to some degree with that which ignited the fear reaction is to have recognized it as belonging to nature, and thus to us as well. It was frightening because it was seen as alien. When its relatedness to us is recognized, the heart relaxes.

This aspect of the practice becomes particularly significant as we go about our daily lives and experience fresh memories or encounters with those things that formerly frightened us, or whatever the habitual emotional reaction might have been. We find that whereas in the past the attention would immediately go into telling ourselves the familiar stories and believing them, or reacting emotionally to conditioned sensory triggers—"I can't believe he said that!" "That's sooo beautiful, I've gotta have it!"—we now notice: "Here's the feeling of desire; here's the feeling of fear," that's all. And if there is a little space around the feeling, we realize we don't have to follow it blindly.

We also find with practice that once we're able to cultivate some clarity around emotional states, we can develop mindfulness of the body to sustain this. When something causes an emotional reaction of any kind to be launched, we can bring the attention into the body and notice where we're feeling it: Where is this anger lodged? This is anticipation, where is this felt? Here's nostalgia, is it hot or cool?

Rather than suppressing or dissociating from the experience in an unskillful way, we are feeling, receiving it fully, but we take the option not to buy into it blindly. The body is thus our means of attuning to the moment, and through its medium we cultivate a responsivity, rather than blind reactivity, to the way things are. This also gradually allows us to "hear" the body's signals before they become screams! This is extremely useful when practicing Yoga as well—to prevent injury, and establish a mindful practice in motion.

Mother Nature's Valium

There is a final element of this practice that derives, again, from the deeply interrelated nature of the physical and mental dimensions of our being.

Say, continuing the example, that you enter a room and someone with whom you have recently had an argument is there. On seeing them a feeling of anxiety arises, accompanied by the thought "Oh no, they're here. What am I going to say to them?"

You have already been working with this kind of reaction for some time, so the mind does not follow with its usual line of thinking: "It's my fear problem again! When am I ever going to be rid of it?" Instead there arises the mindful reflection, "Rather than 'I have a fear problem,' what's really happening here is simply the experience of anxiety arising. It feels like this."

You then consciously bring your attention into your solar plexus area as you walk into the room and notice what physical sensations are there. There is an immediate awareness that your belly has tightened up. You note this and accept it, and then you allow the next natural out-breath to be accompanied by a deliberate softening of the area. There is a tangible relaxation as you let the muscles loosen.

Once that relaxation has been effected, you take a moment to ask yourself, "Now, what was that that I was worried about?" To your surprise, the thinking mind stumbles, gropes for a moment to recall what the big issue was. This is the clue to the true source of worry: it's almost impossible to sustain a good fret if your belly is not tight. When the memory of the argument resurfaces, and those old tapes begin to replay in your thoughts, you bring attention to your solar plexus once again and—lo and behold—it's as tight as a drum. So you relax again. . . .

As you continue into the room and engage with the various people there, particularly when you interact with the other protagonist who sparked the anxiety, you keep part of your attention focused on your body and respond again and again by releasing any return to a state of tension. This serves to keep the heart open and allows the space to be responsive to the moment. To your surprise, the exchanges with the person you were anxious about are oddly open and uncomplicated, honest and without residue. The argument is consigned to the "forgive and forget" file.

The body and mind work like a pair of cisterns connected by a pipe at their base; whatever happens to the water in one affects the levels in the other. Most of us are blithely unaware of the extent to which our moods are affected by our physical habits and vice versa; we do not realize that the two are connected. The kind of practice just described shows us how anxiety, for example, is sustained by tension in the body. When that physical tension is relaxed, it's hard to stay anxious.

This is no new discovery, in fact as well as being ancient wisdom, it is the basis of pharmaceuticals such as Valium. Apparently this drug works through being a muscle relaxant, as opposed to having any mood-altering effect on the central nervous system. By developing this dimension of body awareness and responsivity, we are employing Mother Nature's Valium. The advantage is that this spiritual version is nonaddictive and there is no cost.

Knowing the Body through the Mind

One way of describing this series of practices is "knowing the mind through the body." However, these are by no means the only ways to use meditation on the body and reflective practices to help further the quality of self-understanding and to bring our lives into a more profound state of harmony—far from it.

Jill Satterfield, a colleague I have worked together with on numerous meditation retreats and who runs the Vajra Yoga and Meditation Studio in Manhattan, teaches a practice that might well be named "knowing the body through the mind." It employs a method of visualization, imagining the body as a house.

With an initial injunction to her Yoga students to keep the framework of the exercise "as childlike as possible,"[10] she then walks them through a series of inquiries:

> Where is the brightest room? Where is the darkest?
>
> Which is the most cluttered room?
>
> Where do your parents live when they stay?
>
> Do they ever leave?
>
> Where do you store your childhood memories?
>
> If you could bring in a handyman, what would you ask him to fix?
>
> Which is the coziest, comfiest room?
>
> Would you like to exchange houses with anyone?[11]

She then directs a mindful breathing into the dark or cluttered areas and advises on poses to open and illuminate that part of the body.

As a final element of the exercise she encourages students to self-prescribe restorative poses. These the yogis are guided to choose through visualizing the opening of the windows of their house, throwing out the clutter or, most importantly, through nonfixing of the imperfections but just by sitting close by and being with what is—just as any friend would be with another friend in need.

A Self-Adjusting Universe

A few practices have been spelled out in detail here, and hopefully these descriptions will be of some use, but there's an issue that always comes into play along with the attempt to apply such things in our lives.

In any kind of spiritual discipline, be it Buddhist meditation, Hatha Yoga, Christian prayer, Sufi dancing, or whatever, a perennial problem is that of getting caught in the doing-ness and thing-ness of a tradition or a practice.

We might faithfully follow the formula, putting forth great effort with sincerity, but being guided by the paradigm of "me doing it how it should be done" disappointingly only leads us to depression. We get confused by this and presume that we're just not sincere enough, not trying hard enough, so we crank it all up and pile on more of the "right" thing. We might carry on in this vein for a while, but after some years it can become seriously disheartening.

As a more promising option, we might hunt around and find ourselves a new brand of Buddhism, a new Yoga teacher, or we go back to Christianity, convert to Judaism . . . but after another stint, this starts to pale too. We grasp it all too tightly or we throw it all away—so it goes.

We want to change something in us—all spiritual disciplines are based upon this fact—so this is not the issue. The issue has more to do with the attitude with which we pick up a practice or a tradition than with the particular factors it comprises. What matters is that we find a skillful way of holding it.

Unentangled Participation

The two areas of mishandling in the above paradigm are the "me doing it" and the "how it should be done." We unconsciously create a solid sense of me-ness—known as ahamkara in Pali—along with an equally solid thing that we're trying to do, that is, "my practice." In Pali this quality of mine-ness is known as mamamkara. The more tightly we grasp the "me" and the sense of doing, together with the perceived substantiality and goodness of our "thing"—be it a Yoga āsana, a meditation practice, or our Jewish faith—the more prone we are to disappointment. It is a direct relationship.

So, what to do? We seem to find ourselves straddling both the wisdom of the Third Zen Patriarch, who said, "The faster they hurry, the slower they go," and the wisdom of the Red Queen, who said, "It takes all the running you can do, to keep in the same place."[12]

A way forward is suggested by some of the principles that have already been described here. It is in turning gently away from the habits of either grasping the way things are, on the one hand, or rejecting the way they are, on the other. Instead, being mindful of the natural order of things, the heart attunes itself to the present, and then, through the intrinsic participation of our bodies and minds in the way things are, ways of working fruitfully with the present reality arise spontaneously. We work with the way things are.

It is interesting that, in the Pali language the word for "the truth" is *dhamma* (*dharma* in Sanskrit). In addition to this it also means "duty" or "work, métier." It can also validly be rendered as "nature." This implies that not only are all of our physical and mental attributes part of the entire natural order but also, most significantly, participation is an active, initiative-filled role. We are not disturbing the universe (as T. S. Eliot put it) by responding and choosing. Our free-willed choices are part of "the way things are" and when these choices come not from a self-centered viewpoint, but instead issuing from mindfulness, wisdom, and kindness, the result is joyful and liberating. It is an unentangled participation that leads to peace.

Holding in Awareness

There is a very simple method of viewing this process of unentangled participation in action.

Take some occasion when you are by yourself. It is not crucial that you be sitting in meditation, you could also be standing still or sitting in a chair. The important thing is that you have a few minutes to yourself and can freely turn your attention inward.

Let your mind relax, and do not focus on any particular thing in fact for this purpose. It will help to let your mind wander for a while. After a few minutes bring the attention into the body and sweep it through. You will be sure to notice areas in the body that now seem tight, twisted, slumped, or stressed. Choose the most prominent of these to focus on. Let's say, for instance, this is your spine.

Notice any impulses to straighten those kinks out of your back, but do not act on them. Don't do anything. This is a practice of nondoing, a diligent effortlessness, nonmeditation.

Let the attention settle fully on that crooked feeling in your back and hold it in awareness. Let that holding be as impartial and open as possible: you are not tensing up against it, you are not waiting for it to go away or straighten out, you are not freezing in position—there is a simple and radical acceptance of how it is. You are not wanting it to change. No agenda but awareness.

As you relax into this openhearted awareness, let go of all subtle holdings and controls. Let go of control of the body so that if it wants to move, it can move.

Soon you notice the body starting to make little adjustments—first maybe to one side, then it's still, then way over to the other side. As these little movements occur, don't try to influence them. Rather, leave them alone. Don't try to make them happen. Don't try to make them not happen. Trust in awareness.

Sustain the environment of awareness and simply watch, feel the body changing. Surrender, with faith in the body's own wisdom. Get out of the way. Let the universe adjust itself.

Within a few minutes you find that the body has straightened and the spine is as perfectly aligned as it has ever been. You didn't do anything.

If thoughts arise such as, "Wow! This is great! Now I'm sitting perfectly," let them pass. Or you can try grasping them and identifying with the process, thinking, "Now that I know the trick, I'll really impress the gang at the Yoga studio," and see what happens to that exquisite balance, that perfect natural posture. You'll find that it has changed again.

I often describe this process as "the heat lamp effect." The combination of awareness and radical acceptance (otherwise known as loving-kindness, mettā in Pali) acts like a heat lamp on a knotted muscle; under the influence of those rays all resistance is futile and the knot surrenders, the muscle returns to its natural state in the order of things.

You just lie there while it happens, all you have to do is to receive the heat and let nature take its course. This method of holding in awareness is analogous, although these "rays" are coming from inside.

Practitioners of Hatha Yoga will also be somewhat familiar with this way of working with the mind and body, although it is probably referred to in different ways. In the past I have heard this kind of letting go of self-centered motivation, or nondoing, as "surrendering into the pose," "relaxing into the full expression of a pose" or simply as "getting out of your own way."

In Sanskrit "surrender" is pranidhāna and it is recognized as being a spiritual quality of prime importance. It is the relinquishment of the self-centered perspective; even though at first glance it might seem to have the opposite meaning, ironically, it can be said to be related to the Buddhist concept of faith (saddhā in Pali). For isn't it the case that when the ego surrenders, when we let go of the self-centered view of things, we are, in the same breath, expressing a trust in the fundamental orderliness of nature? We can surrender the urge for control by "me" as we have faith in the infinitely more trustworthy, self-adjusting universe. The result is the inexpressible beauty of full expression.

Jill Satterfield speaks of this kind of selfless full expression of a Yoga āsana as being like origami. The paper surrenders to its folding and unfolding without resistance; the folder lets the fingers make their well-practiced moves, guided simply by these same qualities of kindness and awareness.

She describes the way she uses the metaphor: "The paper is folded into various shapes, then unfolds back into just a piece of paper again, then another shape, then paper again. No matter what the shape, it's still just a piece of paper. No matter what "pose," it's still the body with a potentially clear, uninhibited mind."[13]

The Suchness of the Body

Another curious characteristic of the word *dhamma* is the adjective that derives from it, *dhammatā*, meaning "natural" or "of the nature of ultimate reality." In the Thai language, many of whose words derive directly from Pali terms, and this one has been transmuted into the word *tammadah,* which always means "ordinary," "unremarkable," or "mundane."

This confluence of meanings—"ultimate reality" and "ordinary"—echoes a comparable, if not identical confluence in the word that the Buddha chose to refer to himself: Tathāgata.

The word is made up of two well-known parts, yet scholars have debated for centuries as to what the word was really supposed to mean. Is it *Tath-āgata,* "thus come," or *Tatha-gata,* "thus gone?" "Come to suchness" or "gone to suchness"—which is the real meaning?

The Buddha was very fond of wordplay, however, and my suspicion is that he coined the word *Tathāgata* precisely because it implied both attributes: is that Buddha quality completely transcendent—utterly gone? Or is it immanent in the physical world—completely here, present now? The term is perfect in that it carries both these meanings and indicates that the two, embodiment and transcendence, do not exclude each other in any way.

This attribute of suchness then carries with it the spirit of inclusivity, being the point of intersection of the embodied and the transcendent, of time with the timeless. It directs us toward finding spiritual fulfillment in the suchness of the embodied mind, here and now, rather than in some abstracted, idealized "me," some other place and time, or in a special über-heavenly state we might reach through withdrawal of senses.

When the light of these insights is brought to bear on the interface of Hatha Yoga and Buddhist practice in current times, just as with our heat lamp, we can witness a transforming realization.

As Mary Paffard, another close collaborator and friend of our community who helps run Yoga Mendocino, in Ukiah, California, put it:

> The Yoga is not simply a supplement to an aching back for meditation, and the Buddhism is not just a philosophy of mind divorced from the body . . . it's beyond the two languages and, in the beingness of the body, it comes together.[14]

Maybe if the warmth and brightness of this type of insight is allowed to shine on the Buddhist and Hatha Yoga communities of the West, the universe will be moved to adjust itself and the suchness of body of our spiritual families will be a meeting point for us all.

> In this world of Suchness
> there is neither self, nor other-than-self.
>
> —Seng T'san, *the Third Zen Patriarch, Verses on the Faith Mind*

13

PRACTICE MAPS OF THE GREAT YOGIS

MICHAEL STONE

> The yogi travels from outside to inside and then from inside to outside, just to come to the understanding that outside and inside are not different aspects, but one.
>
> —Swami Lakshmanjoo

It's early dawn, and along with innumerable others who form a syncopated and invisible practice community extending back thousands of years, I quietly make my way to a cleared space to sit still and observe the incoming and outgoing winds of the breath. I light a thin stick of incense, a narrow candle, and though I live in a populated corner of a modern city, I can still make out a glowing morning star.

Two thousand years after the Buddha's instructions on meditative inquiry, and hundreds of years after the fine craftsmanship of the great Japanese poets, and still many more years since the inner cartography laid down by Hatha yogis such as Svātmārāma, I follow their radical inspiration through the practice of Yoga postures, sitting, listening, and learning, as best I can, their elegant maps, codes, and questions. They left behind maps for practice, not doctrine, and it's to these maps I give my attention and inquiry.

Formal Practice Begins

Pressing the sitting bones down into the buckwheat meditation cushion creates the complementary upward action in the spine that gives the rib cage buoyancy and brightness and allows the respiratory diaphragm to move freely. When the pelvis becomes rooted, the skull floats easily and the breath is unlocked—free to come and go. As the breath begins to settle into its natural and irregular rhythm, the nervous system responds, not just chemically but through the visceral sense of fingers becoming still, eyes focusing receptively on the floor in front of crossed ankles, and slowly an entire history of mental and physical activity settles into focused concentration. "Morning," "it's early," "there's a bird," become passing displays of constant thought—arising, collapsing, and irrelevant.

The legs provide a strong base and the spine settles into its natural four-curved ease, and after some time the mind no longer lingers on "leg," "upright," or "breathing out," and the mechanism in the mind that loves labels and a good story slowly fades away. Sitting meditation with focus on the natural and irregular patterns of the breath is a somatic practice. We work with the mind by entering the body. As time rolls on, the concentration invited by this quiet posture begins to open into an all-encompassing awareness that begins in the subtle feelings of in-breathing and extends all the way through the texture of sound and the feel of air both inside and outside the body. Even the city is breathing: streetcars rolling in the distance, seagulls creasing the sky overhead, children late for school, the salaried on their way to work—the earth and community as one shared, animated body. The nervous system quiets down, and patterns of mind and body arise and pass away in the spaciousness of awareness. The world appears with much more clarity than it did when I was caught in ideas and fixations. This is the inner tradition of the great yogis.

The yogin Uddālaka in the medieval collection of Yoga and Buddhist stories the *Yoga Vaśiṣṭa,* describes this succinctly:

> In this body in which there is flesh, blood, bones and organs, who says, "This is what I am, this is me." Motion is the nature of energy and thinking is a pattern of consciousness. This is all free of selfhood. Just as a cloud sitting at the top of a hill does not belong to the hill, I am none of these. So please senses, please body, perform your actions without so much memory.[1]

Even the notion of "body" or the term *air* is irrelevant in deep concentration. Sensations occur in awareness, not simply "in the body." As soon as the mind claims these feelings in terms of a "me" inside a body, they become localized and personal, and we confuse what's occurring in awareness with something that belongs to "I," "me," or "mine." "Leave the body in the body," the Buddha suggests in his teaching in the *Satipaṭṭhānā Sutta* (Establishment of the Foundations of Mindfulness). There is freedom in leaving the body in the body, the breath as the breath, sound as sound, and thought as thought, without picking up every phenomenon and experiencing them as something belonging to "me" personally.

As I tune in to this coming and going of phenomena, from sound to breath to thought, I notice that awareness is stable when the breath relaxes and the body rests in its natural state. In fact, everything of which I am aware is constantly changing, from the images that move through the eyes to the sounds that are perceptible to the ear; even the thoughts that move endlessly through the mind—these are all phenomena of the natural world, constantly materializing and passing away in front of awareness. I need not focus on every thought; instead I can rest in the wisdom that everything is changing and empty of ongoing permanence.

Who Is Breathing?

The breath in Sanskrit is called vāyu, or a wind, and after some time, the breath feels as impersonal as wind and the sensations that once distracted me—a pain in the lower back, an itch on the scalp—also become impersonal phenomena moving through awareness. Whether in seated meditation or in the deliberate and expansive movements of Yoga postures, not only does change seem clear, but I also notice the way any interference in this process on the part of the mind interrupts this internal silence and gives rise to elaborative ideas and imaginings that serve to distract me from the profound and simple gesture of paying attention to what is. I feel connected to something greater than my stories about myself, and after years of practice this attention can be sustained for longer periods of time.

I hear a bird in the distance and immediately an image forms in the mind's eye of a blue jay, and the mind in its naming of "blue jay" already has a historical narrative formed about the blue jay, which I assume to be similar to the one that breezed through my backyard yesterday. Thinking about yesterday pulls me away from the sounds *now,* and slowly I feel unease again. The mind seems like a muscle that contracts around every object of awareness, turning it into something known and understood, even if what I perceive is incorrect. These linguistic moves of the mind are rooted in the past. But "the past" does not exist; the past is simply what the mind is doing in present experience. How the mind remembers, and what the body recalls, may be residue from past impressions, but the movement of content into awareness is *not* historical, it is happening now.

The mind-body process is constantly receiving and shape-shifting what we experience, yet the mind's governing banner is everywhere to be seen, leading to a confusion or misidentification of the names we have for things with life itself. I think the breath is happening in my very own body, but on closer inspection the breath is just occurring, sensations are also occurring, and without the concept "my body" the experience unfolds without boundary or context, and as this concentration is sustained, a previously unknown form of awareness surfaces that includes everything. Sounds and texture, like thought and image, come and go in the same way everything else comes and goes, and for a period of time I am not dominated by a mode of cognition that always compares one thing to another. The conceit of "I am" falls away and an infinite freedom emerges. This is the freedom to be no one. At a visceral level, the experience is characterized by stillness, vitality, and a sense of intimacy with everything, and this entire process begins in the body.

House Builder

Dōgen confirms our addiction to the delusion that "knowing about things" is actual contact with how things are:

> That the self that advances and confirms the myriad things is called delusion
>
> That the myriad things advance and confirm the self is called enlightenment.[2]

What motivates us to step out of the habits and certainties of our lives and the seemingly secure shelter of pleasure and knowledge, and instead move deeper into the world, not by confirming reality with names and ideas but through a simple disappearing act—exchanging a life dominated by self-image for a life immersed in the ordinary natural world? At first such a quest must seem idealistic: can we truly leave behind self-conceit and press our habits into something observable and transformable so that we can return to our basic wholeness? When we focus in on the very small micro-movements of the breath and sensations of the body, we hone our attention on something so small that we are able to study it in detail. Although what we are looking at seems like a microcosm at first, it opens into the wider world of life itself. When I focus in on the shifting patterns of the breath, I am tuning in to the subjective experience of the entire universe.

In Buddhist terminology, practice aims toward nirvāṇa, which literally means "to blow out" or "extinguish." Nirvāṇa is not a final state or holy utopia but rather what is left when craving (tanhā) is relinquished. Because our suffering and lack (duḥkha) is rooted in craving and incessant wanting, when these habits of desire come to an end, self-conceit also comes to an end. We start small, even with the breath, and through sustained attention to the breath we yoke body and mind into quietude and calmness. This process allows discursive throught to fall away. What disappears through the concentric process of awakening is the constant momentum of craving and its associated symptoms of greed, ill will, and delusion. This is where the Buddha begins his formal practice.

In describing how the mind organizes reality, the Buddha suggests that the birth and rebirth of each and every moment is characterized by suffering when perception is dominated by craving. And whenever the mind is not at ease, we are held captive by self-image. Attempting to go beyond his own ideas about the mind and reality, the Buddha looks deeply into his own mind but finds it difficult to investigate his life clearly. "Seeking but not finding the builder of the house" the Buddha sits still under the old ashvattha tree (*Ficus religiosa,* the Indian fig) and begins paying attention to the turbulent movement of thoughts and the workings of body in order to see how they operate *as they are,* independent of his notions and expectations. Like yogis before him, the Buddha intuited that the only way to know the nature of things is to sit still and investigate from a place of quietude. The natural world, as manifest in the body, is the perfect place to begin.

After six years of concentrated meditation and questioning, the Buddha proclaims the freedom that comes from looking and listening deeply to the workings of the mind and seeing through the conceit of "I am" that dominates our perceptions:

> I traveled through the rounds of countless births,
> seeking but not finding the builder of this house.
> Sorrowful is birth again and again.
> O Housebuilder, you have been seen,

you will not build this house again.
Your rafters have been broken,
your ridgepole shattered.
My mind has attained the unconditioned,
achieved is the end of craving.[3]

Radical Questioning

It's so hard for us to learn how to work with the mind body process, because most of the time we are caught in habits of thought and concept. Once the Buddha realizes that he has found the cause of suffering in his own mind, he decides to look no further. Instead, through focusing on the nature of reality as it presents itself in each and every moment—whether through thought, image, fantasy, sensation, or feeling—the Buddha realizes that his mind and body are simply human manifestations of the natural world.

By seeing through the conditioning of the mind—symbolized by house building—Gautama Buddha begins to experience himself as a movement of life itself. Like the yogis before and after him, rather than turning to ritual or scripture, the Buddha relied on his own subjective investigation of mind, body, and the natural world as the point of entry on his path toward freedom. The body and breath, like the morning star, are not symbols or metaphors or something to go beyond, but rather the present manifestation of the truth. Nothing is hidden!

For ancient yogis, the answers provided by ritual worship, religious doctrine, or the priestly classes did not satisfy these existential dilemmas, which proved too magnetic and important to simply be ignored. In fact after the Vedic period of ancient India, forest dwellers and wanderers began to emerge along the Ganges Valley. These were people for whom the reliance on gods and ritual did not secure transcendence or enlightenment. Freedom from discontent and lack did not come from established answers; in fact, the answers provided by the culture-at-large seemed to repress the deepest question of having been born and having to die and somehow having to make meaning of a life structured by death. Can the gods save us from ourselves? Is there a path that transforms the psychological, physiological, and cultural habits that keep the mind spinning in habitual cycles of thought and disorientation? Describing his experience of alienation, the narrator of the early *Ṛg Veda* declares, "I do not know who or what I am. I wander about concealed and wrapped in thought."[4]

What should I do with this fleeting life? Why do I feel separate from those around me and why is relief from existential anxiety so brief and momentary? How do I work with all the habits in my mind so that I can tune in to the nature of reality rather than my self-created ideas about those around me and the inner and outer world I inhabit?

To understand the emergence and depth of the various traditions of Yoga and Buddhism, it's best to begin with questions that give rise to contemplative inquiry. Like all the great spiritual traditions, both Yoga and Buddhism were born within particular cultural conditions, and those conditions informed the way one sought to investigate the great matters of life and death, but what characterizes the Yoga of the Buddha is that the spiritual path begins not only with a recognition of duḥkha but also with rigorous questioning rather than answers. Instead of beginning the path with theories of creation or stories of omnipotent gods, the Buddha encourages inquiry and attention to the here and now.

While wandering in the Kosala country with a large community of bhikkhus, the Buddha entered a town of the Kalama people. The Kalamas paid homage to the Buddha and asked for guidance in practice, particularly in understanding where to put their faith. The Buddha responded,

> "Come, Kalamas. Do not go upon what has been acquired by repeated hearing; nor upon tradition; nor upon rumor; nor upon what is in a scripture; nor upon surmise; nor upon an axiom; nor upon specious reasoning; nor upon a bias towards a notion that has been pondered over; nor upon another's seeming ability; nor upon the consideration, 'The monk is our teacher.' Kalamas, when

you yourselves know: 'These things are good; these things are not blamable; these things are praised by the wise; undertaken and observed, these things lead to benefit and happiness,' enter on and abide in them."[5]

In a culture where ritual and organized worship dominated the landscape of religious inquiry, yogis left the villages and temples and moved into the unfamiliar territory of forests and plains, uninhabited river deltas and quiet natural retreats. Although our historical eyes tend to idealize the quietude of such surroundings, the archetypal nature of the yogi's quest is more important than historical guesswork or romanticism. What we know from the surviving practices and teachings is that what we call "a yogi" is someone who turned inward to discern the nature of life, the life of the mind, and how even the notions of "inward" and "outward" are products of the mind. When we look inward or outward, we find mind and body in all manifestations, since we cannot observe or perceive the world without the sense organs (body-mind) and consciousness.

In another passage, from the *Canki Sutta,* the Buddha describes hearing the dharma with one's whole body, reflecting on it, studying it, and not taking truth to be something expressed by somebody else:

> Having heard the Dharma, he [the student] memorizes it and examines the meaning of the teachings; when he has gained a reflective acceptance of those teachings, zeal springs up; when zeal has sprung up, he applies his will, he scrutinizes . . . he realizes with the body the supreme truth and sees it by penetrating it with wisdom. In this way . . . there is the discovery of truth.[6]

Nothing Is Hidden

One of the characteristics of the teachings of great yogis such as Siddhartha Gautama, Patañjali, Nagarjuna, Dōgen, and others is that they show us that traditional and institutionalized forms of religion and ritual are not the only way to the truth. At some point we must sit still and pay attention. Lineage, adherence to a particular school, or complete obedience to saṅgha, do not guarantee access to the truth.

Perhaps what Yoga and Buddhist teachings share is a radical challenge to the way in which we conceive of spirituality. They do this by reorienting our metaphysical and spiritual quest so that we do not look for meaning or transcendence somewhere hidden from view or waiting for us in another lifetime. Instead *transcendence* is reinterpreted as "immanence," allowing us to wake up to the transient nature of our lives and the way that craving and wanting obscure our true nature. For both Yoga and Buddhism, the path that orients the practitioner toward present experience begins right here, right now, in this body, at this time.

The Buddha, like Patañjali, did not create a new system of practice; but rather, he pointed out what's already present. The radical Buddhist philosopher Nagarjuna wrote,

> When buddhas don't appear
> And their followers are gone
> The wisdom of awakening
> Bursts forth by itself.[7]

"The wisdom of awakening" depends on a mind free of entanglements and distractions, free to think and wonder and see clearly. All Nagarjuna is doing, writes radical Christian theologian Don Cupitt,

> is simply stating the obvious—spelling out clearly and consistently what is implied by the recognition that everything in our experience, and everything within ourselves too, is contingent and changing. And similarly, Buddhists normally insist on the importance of lengthy training under the guidance of a recognized teacher from a strong lineage; but Nagarjuna is saying that the central Buddhist insight [to] completely accept universal contingency and transience, within and without, is bliss—and

this thought is so easy to come at that it may occur to anyon
any time.[8]

Waking up, Gautama reminds us, is not dependent on anything outside of our mind. "It is as if electricity disappeared from the face of the earth," writes Zen teacher John Daido Loori,

> . . . and someone, a billion years from now, created a generator, started turning it, and coiled a wire and attached it to the generator; the more they turned the hotter the wire would get until finally it glowed and light appeared. It would be the same light now produced by light bulbs, the same electricity. All they would have to do is produce the electricity. In the case of the Buddhadharma, all that needs to be done is to realize it. What do you realize? What you realize is that Buddha mind has always been here. You do not attain it, you were born with it. Zen did not come to America from Japan; it was always here and will always be here.[9]

Like Nagarjuna's comment about the "wisdom of awakening bursting forth," John Daido Loori reminds us of the inherent awakened nature in all things. The Buddha did not quarrel with other schools nor did he attempt a philosophical or metapsychological framework for his teaching. He taught different things to different people at different times, not because his ideas changed but because we all need different pointers. Again, what unites the traditions of Yoga and Buddhism is not the similarities between terms or lists or metaphors but the fact that there is no tradition, path, or self to be defended or reified.[10] Even when we begin to characterize Buddhism as the Four Noble Truths, the *Wisdom Heart Sūtra* negates such reification every step of the way: "No suffering, no source, no relief, no path."[11]

Though I teach students in a small community in Toronto, and though we follow the maps outlined in the *Hatha Yoga Pradīpika,* the *Yoga Sūtra,* and other ancient texts, I always remind students that we must embody these practices and express them in our lives, not rely completely on the written word. The dharma is passed along through its expression in our lives, not through mimicking what the elders have taught. A map is only useful if it comes to life in the present landscape. We change the maps as we practice with them. Practice, even when rooted in tradition, is a living, changing, breathing organism.

These teachings present an uncompromising challenge for each and every one of us to engage the potential within us to actualize the teachings presented. There is no security available in the world of things, and every move we make to contract around that which is ultimately fleeting returns us to the wheel of saṃsāra—a conditioned existence—which is nothing other than a metaphor for meaninglessness. The anxiety that letting go provokes points us toward existential questions that will not go away. The great yogis can't do it for us, neither can texts or doctrine or ritual. We must use the reality of our everyday experience in mind and body to see through the carapace of a life of habit and self-centeredness. How can we serve others if we are always filtering the world through "I, me, and mine"?

Practice Is the Way

When the Buddha sat down to watch his own breath, he knew that no insight was possible until his mind was settled and his body was at ease. Such ease allowed him to study the nature of reality, and he began with the incoming breath and outgoing breath and the feeling of being in a body. In his teaching on the Four Foundations of Mindfulness, the Buddha instructs,

> Breathing in a long breath, he [the practitioner] knows, "I am breathing in a long breath"; breathing out a long breath, he knows, "I am breathing out a long breath."
>
> Breathing in a short breath, he knows, "I am breathing in a short breath"; breathing out a short breath, he knows, "I am breathing out a short breath."[12]

Notice how the Buddha tunes us in to the feelings of breathing in the body without worrying if the breath needs to be a certain way or if the body is healthy, skinny, old, or young. "Look at the blossoms and also the decay," he seems to be saying. "Watch the entirety of the breath cycle from beginning to end, one after the next." When I teach this to my students, I interpret these initial instructions as follows:

> If you feel the breath is short, no need to make it long.
> If you feel the breath is long, no need to make it short.
> Let the breath even itself out; let it be inconsistent and natural.
> Feel the breath as it's materializing without adding anything to it.

The Buddha is not pointing out a Divine Source of Life but rather attentiveness to the here and now of contingent experience. Whatever is occurring, we pay attention without judgment and the wonderful thing about meditating on the body is that as we release tension patterns or habitual holding schemas, the hologram of the body and mind begin to release one another, because they are interwoven. Dense constrictions in the physical body carry associated feelings and emotions that are, in turn, punctuated by stories, memories, and concepts. Can we feel and listen to the breath and its natural movement without changing it in any way? As the breath settles, so too does the mind; when we are caught in physical holding patterns, the mind's ideas about those sensations must also be released, or the karmic patterns of aversion continue to roll on both physically, mentally, and emotionally. Mind and body are two ends of the same stick.

This assertion is illustrated in case 20 from the Zen *Book of Serenity:*

> Let it be short, let it be long—stop cutting and patching; Going along with the high, along with the low, it levels itself. Not knowing is nearest.[13]

"Not knowing" is a Zen term that describes openness of mind and flexibility of perception and is not necessarily the opposite of knowing. Not knowing is the state of mind in which awareness observes what's occurring without being entangled in preferences, oppositions, likes, or dislikes. Not knowing is the open awareness occurring when we give up fixed ideas about ourselves and others. Whether the breath is short or long, or sensations materializing in the body are pleasant or painful, awareness absorbs what is occurring and allows these patterns to level themselves off on their own. Can we drop into the felt sense of the body vacant of stories and frames? Patañjali's well-known sūtra on the practice of āsana sounds quite similar:

> The postures of meditation should embody steadiness and ease.
> This occurs as all effort relaxes and coalescence arises, revealing that the body and the infinite universe are indivisible.
> Then one is no longer disturbed by the play of opposites.
>
> With effort relaxing, the flow of inhalation and exhalation can be brought to a standstill; this is called breath regulation.
> As the movement patterns of each breath—inhalation, exhalation, lull—are observed as to duration, number, and area of focus, breath becomes spacious and subtle.
> As realization dawns, the distinction between breathing in and breathing out falls away.
> Then the veil lifts from the mind's luminosity.[14]

Notice how Patañjali includes the postures of both meditation (āsana) and breath regulation (prāṇāyāma) as techniques that point toward a release of effort, not just physically but mentally—a release that reveals the nondual nature of reality free from opposites of "me" and "my body" or even "inhaling" and "exhaling." Life flows, birds fly, fish swim. The body knows how to breathe. All technique helps release the conditioning that obscures this natural Yoga, this basic intimacy. When these opposites fall away, the veil "lifts from the mind's luminosity," revealing that "the body and the universe are indivisible." The indivisible reality is what we call Yoga, the union of all things before the mind splits the world up into "this" and "that." The breath, like words and opinions, leaks away and never returns again in exactly the same way. Cells and thoughts regenerate moment after moment, flowing though awareness like waves breaking delicately behind each new perception. "I've watched the breath over and over again," the Buddha is reported to have said, "and though I cannot tell you what I've gained, I can tell you what I've lost." The Buddha did not discover anything new and did not claim to have done so. What he woke up to is what you and I can wake up to. Frames of body and mind drop away, and life shows up.

Body and Mind Drop Away

Seng T'san's early Ch'an poem "Relying on Mind" refines the notion that when we tune deeply in to the workings of the body, the witness that I call "me" actually drops away and the body and mind become nothing other than the seamless continuity of the natural world. This occurs when effort releases.

> Suppressing activity to reach stillness
> just creates agitation.
> Dwelling in such dualities,
> how can you know identity?
> People who don't know identity
> bog down on both sides—
> rejecting form, they get stuck in it,
> seeking emptiness, turn away from it.
> The more people talk and ponder,
> the further they spin out of accord.
> Bring grabbing and speculation to a stop,
> and the whole world opens up to you.[15]

The term *accord* refers here to seeing or being with things as they truly are. I always remind my students that Yoga posture practice does not mature by adding more and more spectacular postures but rather through tuning in to things as they happen, via patterns of sensation and breathing that are always present. Any spiritual practice motivated by striving just reinforces craving and self-identity, the two features that give rise to duḥkha (pervasive dissatisfaction).

For many of us, there are areas in the body, as well as deep emotions, that are dormant or stagnant. The practice of prāṇāyāma and āsana are designed to wake up the internal body and bring intelligence and vitality to the whole system of our being until the breath, the nervous system, and the elaborations of the imagination begin to settle. The abbot of a Zen monastery recently attended one of my retreats and commented, "There are movements I practiced that brought me into such untouched areas in the body that I could barely handle the emotions there, particularly the shame that came up that I have not worked with in my zazen. But then I was able to work with that thought. These practices—Yoga postures and zazen [seated meditation]—are of equal value. They illuminate wholly different aspects of mind and body. Both are needed to open me up to the world."

Yoga postures including the variations of sitting still (padmāsana, svastikāsana, virāsana) are all complex patterns of meditative inquiry. The *Netra Tantra* describes this internal form of āsana as follows:

> On the pathway of your breath, maintain continuously refreshed and full awareness on, and in the center of, the breathing in and breathing out. This is force and this is internal āsana.[16]

Through the inhaling (prāṇa) and exhaling (apāna) patterns, we focus the mind on the movement of sensation and breathing until the force of concentration begins to resolve opposites. Technique falls away and the inner alignment of āsana spreads out through the whole body-mind process, revealing an inherent interconnection with all things. The outer techniques of Yoga postures orient the practitioner toward this internal alignment that is as much psychological as it is physical. This is where āsana comes alive.

When we read the old texts on Yoga postures, we find descriptions of the internal pathways of the breath, not the angular or external geometric alignment instructions of contemporary āsana form. Instead we hear about the ways the mind and breath move together through the internal pathways, as expressed in the meridians (nāḍīs) that run through the subtle body. The various Yoga postures are designed to recirculate, stimulate, and balance the energy moving through the mind-body process. The old images of Yoga postures also focus on the quality of the eyes, particularly illustrating receptive gazing (dṛṣṭi) and inward focus (pratyāhāra). Unlike the muscular shapes of modern Yoga photographs, the body appears subtle and at ease, the postures noble and elegant.

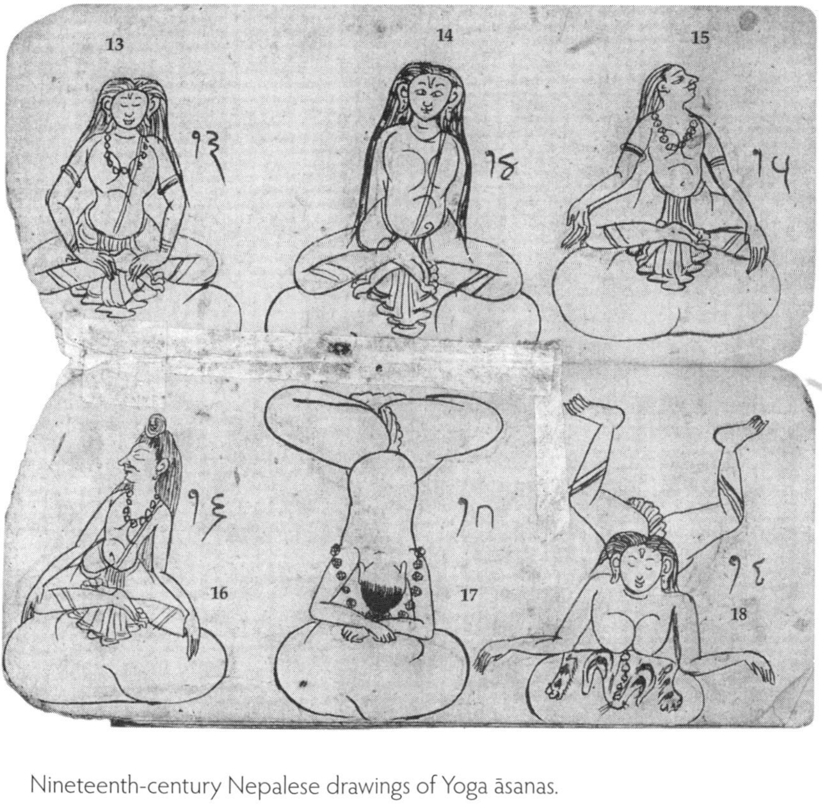

Nineteenth-century Nepalese drawings of Yoga āsanas.

The nāḍīs (rivers, or conduits, of energy) flow from the energetic channels of the spine right out through the body and into the world. The prāṇa (breath energy) flows along with the mental patterns through these internal pathways. This metaphoric language allows us to feel the internal pathways of the breath so that we can settle the mind and nervous system.

Tantra and True Nature

In the tantric traditions of India, China, and Tibet, we find yogis turning their own bodies into places of pilgrimage and mapping out the energetic channels (nāḍīs), platforms (cakras), psychophysical points of meditation (bandhas), and other features of the mental, emotional, and physical landscape. Anyone who follows the breath in seated or moving meditation practices knows that entering the body is like entering a deep forest of unknown territory. There are places the breath flows smoothly and where the mind can remain steady, and there are other centers in the body where there is agitation, strong emotion, or frenzied mental distraction. The tantrikas traditionally described the mind and body in an energetic language that attempts to capture the middle place of mental and physical processes. Sometimes the body is described as container, landscape, mountain range, inverted mountain, river system, energetic axis, net, serpent, or any of the animals that constitute familiar Yoga postures.

From the tantric maps we learn that the exhaling breath (apāna) completes itself in the pelvic floor and the incoming breath (prāṇa) then grows from the center of the pelvic floor (mūla bandha) and up through the central axis (suṣumna nāḍī) of the body. This poetic language attempts to capture the feeling of the breath and what happens in the mind when the endless fog of distraction begins to clear. The mind and body are inseparable twins animated by the breath. Tantric techniques both prior to and after the Buddha focused on tuning in to the subtle energetic movements of body and mind as a means of knowing the ultimate reality beyond egoic "knowing." Valuing feeling and the body, Tantra returns the practitioner to the site of the body over and over again in order to concentrate the mind and realize samādhi (integration).

When we look closely at the transient appearances of body and mind, it is hard to find any one thing that belongs to "I, me, or mine." Even the breath that sustains us is an impermanent wind blowing through the mind-body process with unevenness and an expiry date. Hatha Yoga texts refer to the breath as a series of five winds (prāṇa vāyu), the meridians of the body as flowing rivers (nāḍī), the pelvic diaphragm as the center of the earth (mūla bandha), and the core of the body's axis (suṣumnā nāḍī) as a holy inverted mountain (Mount Meru). Throughout hundreds of years, the internal energetic pathways of the body were mapped and remapped so that yogis can follow a reliable path along which they can feel the subtle movements of mind and body as concentration deepens and wisdom arises. Yoga postures were not forms of exercise as much as they were genuine pathways of liberation.

The breath and emotions tend to become more concentrated in certain areas along the central axis of the body, and over the centuries those platforms (cakras) were given various names so that the yogins could stop along the upward movements of the spine and focus on the energetic, emotional, and psychological holding patterns that occurred there. These maps allowed the yogis to focus on these energetic places so as to bring presence to the internal holding patterns that prevented breath flow and attentiveness. It's not so much that these cakras are literal places but rather that they are tools or lenses through which we can gain a clear understanding and experience of the movements of mind and breath. Sometimes the cakras themselves would be replaced with images of an expanded body containing the entire world of community, family, animals, and devotional icons. What was thought of as a world "outside" becomes the body-world without separation. The "world" is not separate from you.

One of the insights we can explore in Yoga postures is the way the natural world *is* the very body itself. The image below portrays the āsana itself as the place where world and self meet, revealing the nondual

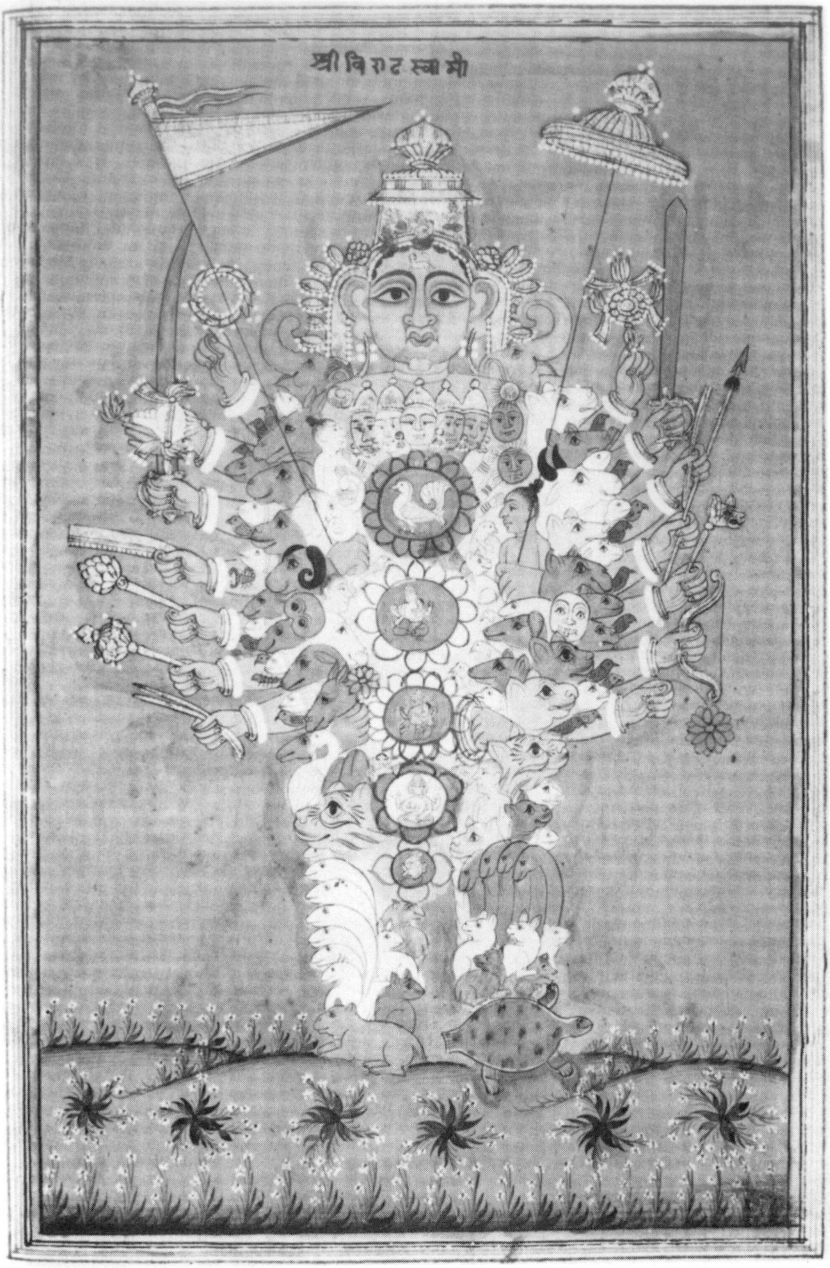

Nineteenth-century Indian drawing of the cosmic form of Viṣṇu-Kṛṣna with cakras of the subtle body during Yoga āsana practice.

functioning of both. The construction of a "world out there" simultaneously creates a "self in here," and this discord is called duḥkha. Yoga reminds us that the biosphere is not something out there but rather the functioning of the breath and body and mind in this very moment.

Each sequence of Yoga postures creates patterns of sensation that in turn loop through the nervous system and give rise to changes in the breath. The poses are designed to stretch our mind's spectrum of preference so that we come to feel our way into the depth of the body without attachment (rāga) or aversion (dveṣa). The breath is then brought into the Yoga pose to accompany sensations as they materialize. By smoothing out the fluctuations of the breath cycle, one also allows the awareness to steady and to enter the primary pathways of the subtle body. Attention (citta) and the energy of the breath (prāṇa) are seen to be two sides of the same coin and slowly they synchronize and clear the internal channels for deep meditative concentration (samādhi) and wisdom (prajñā).

Some illustrations of Yoga postures are so geared toward the inner experience of the practitioner that the internal pathways are depicted without the image of a body at all. When the eyes are closed, as we visualize the breath and feel the movements of energy and emotions in silence, we touch energy centers that have nothing at all to do with the outer form of the body. The image of the outside of the body is replaced with a deep level of attentive feeling.

In this image, the details of the cakras (internal energy centers) are depicted without the human form in the diagram below. The human form then returns in the shape of an āsana (posture) or mudrā (seal or gesture) where the physical body has dropped away in favor of an expanded human form.

Sometimes the details of the illustration serve as guidelines as to how to practice or what kind of feeling may emerge in specific locations. For example, when we look at the map of the mūladhara cakra (root-place

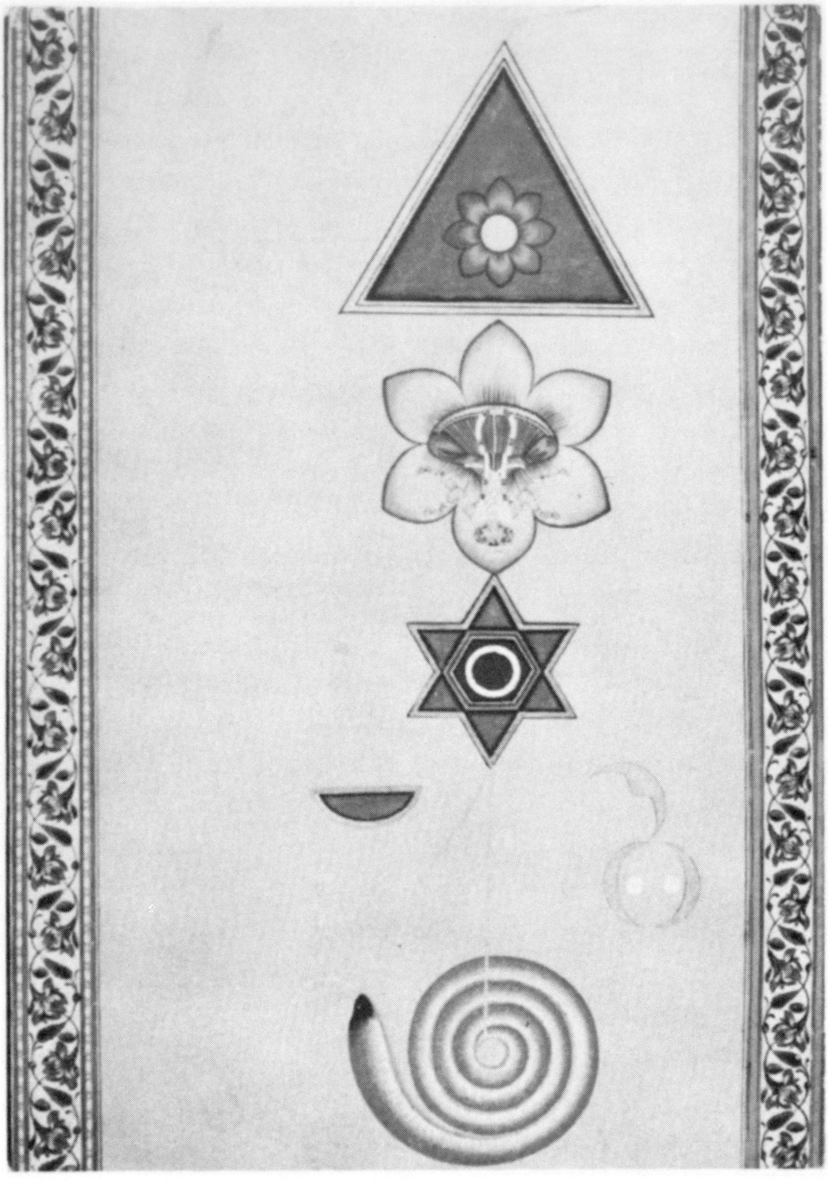

One of seven nineteenth-century Indian paintings of the meditation on the cakras, which together once formed a continuous scroll representing the mind free of all clinging.

diaphragm), also known as mūla bandha (rooted bond), we learn that this can be felt in the pelvic floor at the completion of an exhale. As the exhalation nears its natural pause, the pubic bone, coccyx, and sitting bones point toward one another in a natural skeletal movement. When the pubic bone and coccyx draw toward each other, the pubic-coccygeal muscle and pelvic diaphragm tone in the shape of a circular maṇḍala. These four skeletal corners are represented by the shifted square that surrounds the image. Around that square we find the circular diaphragm (bandha, cakra) of the pelvic floor. Within this image we see an elephant with seven tusks that represents the earth element. Feeling the end of the exhale is considered to be a grounding practice, and most beginning Yoga-posture sequences are forward bends, which force the exhale to a completion point. Many advanced prāṇāyāma exercises train the practitioner to feel the pause at the end of the exhale for long periods of time as an "earthy" and grounding practice. The seven tusks of the elephant represent the seven minerals, which are the essence of the grounding quality of the earth. One meditates on this image as the breath is exhaled and tone appears in the pelvic floor, or a practitioner visualizes this image while chanting seed mantras in order to ground the mind in the core of the body.

Illustration of Moolādhara cakra for visualization as described in *Yoga Cudamami Upaniṣad.*

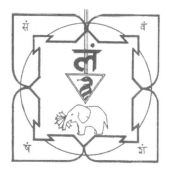

Hatha Yoga, like all forms of Tantra, describes the physiology and feeling tone of human experience, and as such, the metaphors vary from tradition to tradition. Some schools describe energy in terms of kundalini, some in terms of prāṇa devata (the goddess of prāṇa), and others in terms of drops of nectar (bindu/amṛta) that emerge when the mind is in deep absorption and the body is at complete ease. We always need metaphors to speak of deep feelings, so Tantra Yoga is characterized by a colorful mythology. The characters and colors, spinning wheels and internal deities, are all perspectives through which we can enter the wellspring of the mind-body process in order to "touch enlightenment with the body."[17] The body is always a convergence of our lives right now, because it's plastic. Our body and mind are plastic in the sense that they are newly molded in each and every moment in our interactions and can never return to the same form they were in any previous moment in the same way. They are plastic in the sense that when a sculptor creates a form out of a square of marble, it cannot be turned back into the original square again. We are neuronally and socially plastic. By definition, psychological change, spirituality, and ethical action become one and the same when we see the relationship between our motivations, actions, and the effects of our choices. Like the Buddha, when Patañjali points out the mental sequences that give rise to suffering, he lays a foundation for ethical practices based on the understanding that our actions make a difference in the mental stream, the nervous system, and the body politic.

In many schools, the body would be placed into animal shapes so as to leave the human world altogether and enter the natural world through the imagination. Disorienting the mind and disorganizing tension patterns, these shapes were the most popular Yoga poses. They were not designed as a performance but rather as a shamanistic exploration of the internal workings of mind and body in order to become free of the personal patterns that obscure free and easy awareness. Modern Yoga classes are full of these postures.

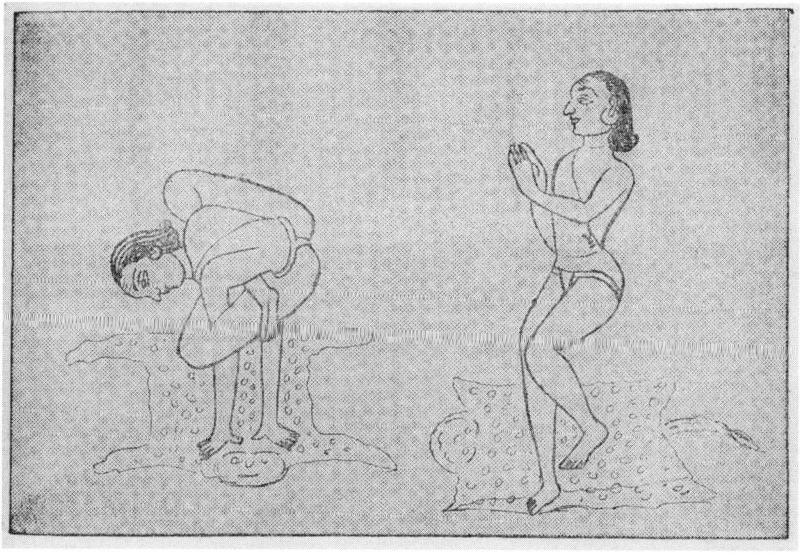

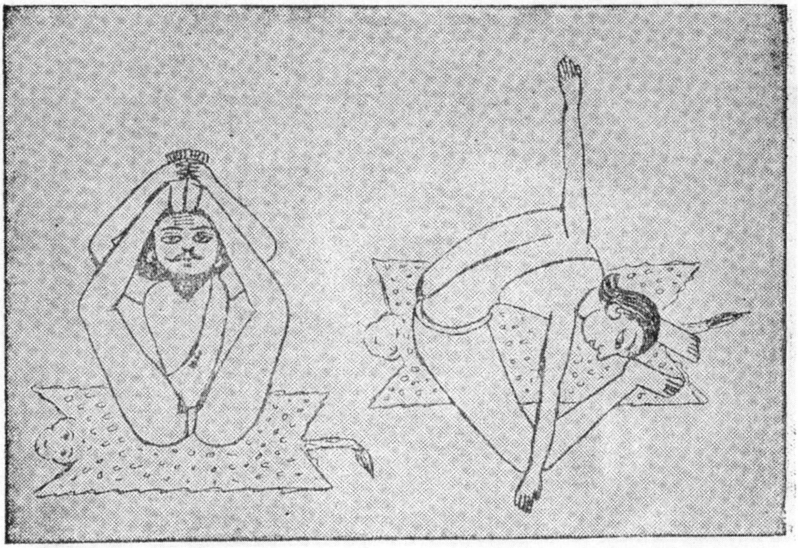

Nineteenth-century Nepalese drawings of Yoga āsanas.

Right Mind, Right Body

As the body becomes pliable and the breath moves freely and intelligently, our thoughts no longer get hooked into old patterns, and we are free to respond to the world without preconceived notions of "me" and "the world." We enter into the Yoga postures not to complete some perfected image or gesture but rather to wake up the intelligent union of mind, body, and heart. Takuan (1573–1645) reminds us of the immovable wisdom we find here in the body and an awareness that is free from fixation and ambition.

> The Right Mind is the mind that does not remain in one place. It is the mind that stretches throughout the entire body and self.
>
> The Confused Mind is the mind that, thinking something over, congeals in one place.[18]

This kind of simple but direct clarity is echoed in the last line of Svātmārāma's *Hatha Yoga Pradīpikā* as both a pithy instruction on motivation and also a stern warning:

> As long as the Prāṇa does not enter and flow through the middle channel of one's mind and body, and the internal energy does not become stable by the control of the movements of prāṇa; as long as the mind does not rest in the ease of the inherent resolution of opposites without any effort, so long all the talk of knowledge and wisdom is nothing but the nonsensical babbling of a madman.[19]

The *Hatha Yoga Pradīpikā* comes to completion with a description of awakening as a mind at ease and a body dynamic and intelligent. Leading up to this passage the author describes the splitting open of the moon and nectar dripping through the palate and into the central axis. Described as immortal bliss (amṛta) or as compassion (karuṇā), the central channel opens and the middle path is realized.

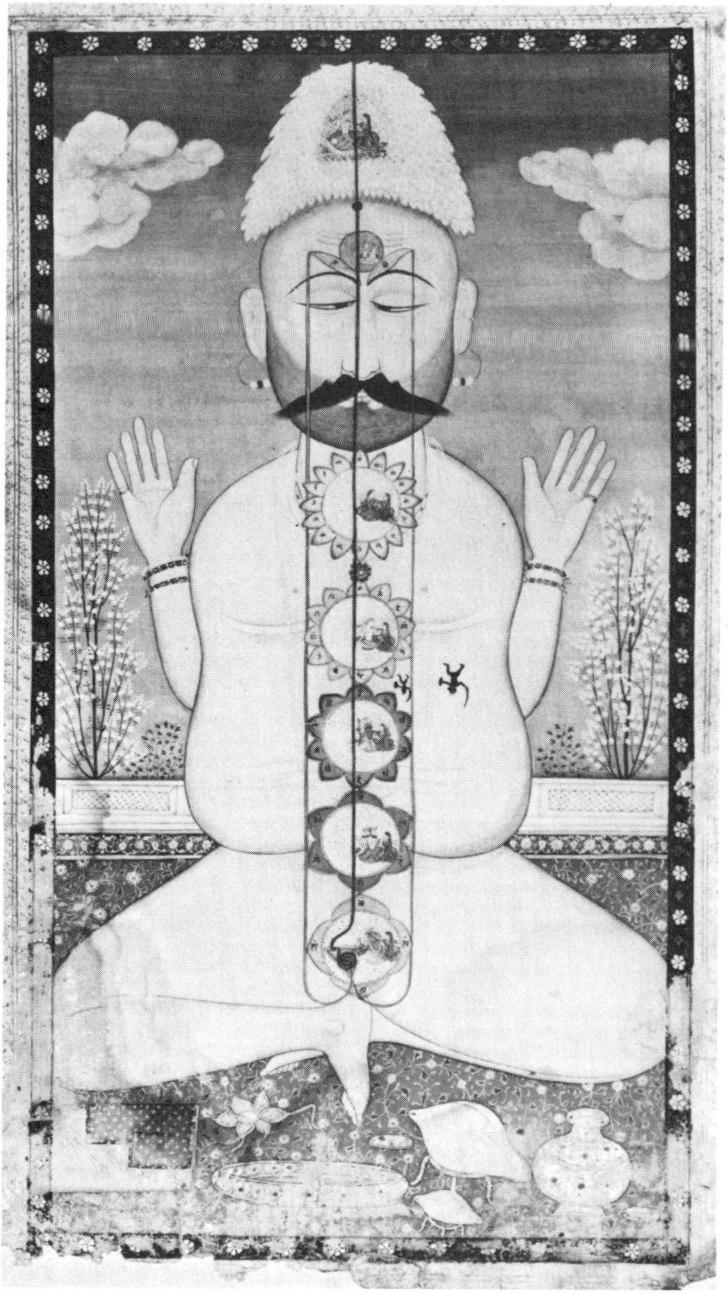

Eighteenth-century Indian diagram of the six cakras in the subtle body.

The Quest

We return always to the body, the breath, and the visceral sense of being alive right here and right now. Being conscious of myself means that I see I have no end and no beginning. "It is not necessary, therefore," writes Chip Hartranft in his commentary on the *Yoga Sūtra,* "to conceptualize, verbalize, or 'make sense' of the meditative experience in order to achieve freedom."[20] In this line of logic, Hartranft says, we must "demand an answer to the following question: if awareness lies at the core of all experience, who is experiencing the awareness?"[21]

It's hard for the mind to accept that it cannot grasp awareness. The egoic nature of our habits of thinking have a basic dilemma we consistently encounter: pure awareness has no personal qualities and stands behind self-image, not in front of it.

The movement away from the Vedic notions of soul, self, seer, or other terms that describe pure awareness needs to be understood in historical context. After the Vedic period, in which Brahmins, the priestly caste, organized and controlled religious ritual and endeavor, new teachings began to emerge called the *Upaniṣads*. The *Upaniṣads* were at first secret and revolutionary, for they claimed that the essence of all reality—Brahmān—is in everything and everyone. Wherever you look and in everything you do, Brahmān is always present. Brahmān is not a thing or a person or an omnipotent controller, but the ever-abiding counterpart to change. One no longer needed the Brahmin class to secure liberation or religious practice because if Brahmān is everywhere, liberation and spiritual practice are also everywhere and in everything. This change characterized the forests and plains through which Gautama traveled after he left his home in Kapalivatthu.[22]

Reading the Buddha's story in symbolic form gives weight to the archetypal dimension of his story, offering another avenue that grounds his experiences in each and every one of us. The palaces young Siddhartha grew up in and eventually left become symbolic of the way pleasure deludes us and distracts us from being with what is. They remind us of the fact that no amount of money nor any number of servants can protect us from the sufferings of impermanence, pain, old age, and death. Gautama's father, Śuddhodana, king of the Sākyas, symbolizes the fact that others have ideas for us, notions about what our lives should look like, and that these ideas often keep us asleep, infantilized, and without the skills necessary to look deeply into the nature of our reality and discover for ourselves what freedom and happiness truly are.

When we turn to texts such as the *Yoga Sūtra* or the medieval text, the *Yoga Vāsiṣṭha,* the philosophies imparted are not just good stories about imagined characters but maps that help us embody the truths they describe. The *Yoga Sūtra* is your textbook, Rama's quest in the *Yoga Vāsiṣṭha* is your own, the body described in the *Hatha Yoga Pradīpikā* is your own body, with its ribs and caves, distractions and aversions. Again, the teachings that emerge from the Axial Age and onward are not given truths that we are to believe on blind faith but rather suggestions for how to live and descriptions of a path toward freedom from lack. Although one may need a guide to help us along the path, every step of the path is available for those who are willing to sit still and look into the nature of the mind and body. And we don't have to look far—the universal truths available to each one of us are right here in this body, in this life, at this time. Kobun Chino Otogawa Roshi (1938–2002) writes,

> The more you sense the rareness and value of your own life, the more you realize that how you use it, how you manifest it, is all your responsibility. We face such a big task, so naturally we sit down for a while.[23]

Encountering the Forest

Religions and philosophies, like linguistic rules and sentence structures, describe the ways we construct our experience and the stories we like to tell about ourselves and our place in the world. But can stories really describe what we are? If we want to penctrate who we are, if we want to become as unself-consciously human as treeness is to a tree, we must go beyond the mapmaking and security blanket of our stories and open to who and what we are.

The way of the squirrel is to eat acorns late into the fall and hibernate in the winter. The way of the tree is to gather her energy into her central axis each winter and, if lucky enough to be a maple or a birch, to produce the most memorable syrup each spring. What is the way of the human? Who are you?

Such questions, whether the result of the natural world or the wild ecology of the human mind-body process, have been the main thrust of yogis since beginningless time.

Robert Bringhurst writes,

> If you really want to understand the tree, you have to encounter it in the forest. If you want to understand the river, you have to go to the watershed. If you want to understand the story, you have to go beyond it, into the ecosystem of stories.[24]

Patañjali, like the Buddha many years before and Nagarjuna many years later, suggests that we must go beyond the ecosystem of story as well, even for short bursts of time, to where we directly encounter the world of sensation and emotion, thought and image, in each and every moment of experience. And whether we know it or not, every time we practice sun salutations and back bends, headstands and breathing practices, we are inquiring into the vastness of reality as it presents itself in this moment. Don't get caught in the form! Our practice is to go beyond the form of the superficial geometry of Yoga poses and instead look into the vast movements of the natural world we call body or mind. Zen teacher Reb Anderson sums up the practice of sitting zazen in good form as "convert[ing] yourself to bodily awareness."[25]

In ordinary life we are not only (mis)identified with the constant interplay of thoughts, but unself-conscious activity is only a fleeting break in an otherwise continuous flow of thought. What the teachings of great yogis like Buddha remind us—through their creative techniques and counterintuitive logic—is that the mind-body process in no way belongs to an "I, me, or mine." Dualistic language of mind and body, self and object, inside and outside is more than mere rhetoric: practice reminds us that we need to continually resist the temptation to stand outside of experience, and instead become the experience.

When you look into the body, what do you actually see? Pay attention not to what you think you see but to what you actually feel in this very moment. Do you notice how the body is not solid but rather an ongoing process of indefinite and beginningless movements of energy? Can you find repeatable patterns that we call "body" or do you find nothing other than a coming together and coming apart of thoughts, feelings, sensations, and other mental formations? Let awareness pervade the body and we begin to open to the greater world as well—not picking and choosing, but returning again and again to what is.

When we no longer create the distinction of parts and sums, "me" and "not me," we can more fully enter into experience. The mind no longer attempts to control fleeting sensations and images and instead we can let go and abide in present experience. Such clarity of awareness and stillness in the body then leads to a sense that there is work to be done, situations to tend to, and actions to be taken. Once we wake up to the reality of interconnection and interdependence, we see that our actions have an effect and that we can't only commit to stillness, especially since other beings are suffering.

Yoga and the Buddhadharma offer us a profound blueprint for reorienting ourselves toward that which really matters. At the heart of what matters is the reality that everyone aspires to achieve happiness and avoid suffering. Happiness derives not from wealth or progress but from an inner peace, one that each one of us must create by cultivating the most profound human qualities, such as empathy, humility, and compassion, and by eliminating destructive thoughts and emotions such as anger and hatred. But many of us can't sit still during the swells of thoughts or turbulent emotions that move through our minds and bodies.

A framework for ethical action rests on the observation that those whose conduct is ethically positive are happier and more satisfied, and the belief that much of the unhappiness we humans endure is actually of our own making.

We act ethically when we do what we know will bring happiness to others and ourselves. When we act toward others with a deep understanding of the interconnectedness of all life, we recognize that everything we do affects others, that everything we do has a universal dimension. We continue to practice in everything we do, even though waking up can sometimes be followed by shutting down again. Through studying the great texts and poets of long ago and maintaining contact with exacting and inspiring teachers of the present day, perhaps we might carry on the living traditions of the dharma by expressing this timeless wisdom in our everyday lives.

Immovable Wisdom of Body and Mind

Life is not a linear structure. It begins and ends where we enter it. But since we have always been in it, there is no middle or beginning, there is no end or final frame of reference, only this very experience. There is no discord between formal practices of body and mind, everyday activity, speaking, and listening. Special retreats and paths are set up to remind us of this. If we truly absorb the essential message of the yogis of old, it is this: there are no activities outside of practice and there is no accomplishment. A Yoga posture has no final endpoint. Neither does the activity of the mind.

Where does the mind end and the body begin? Where does the body end and the world begin? Just as the naturalist moves through the forest with its vast array of trees and animal life, Yoga practices teach us to move deeply into the subtle mind states and energies that make up what we call "the body." With such an attitude mind and body practices become one.

If this mind and body are in seamless continuity with the world-at-large, including rivers and clouds and the body politic, who is it that wakes up?

ACKNOWLEDGMENTS

THIS BOOK HAD its inception in a quiet alley in the west end of Toronto where, over a period of several years, a community of Yoga and Buddhist practitioners gathered to explore what spiritual practice means for them outside the organized form of the temple, zendo, sanctuary, or commercial Yoga studio. Eventually we gave the community the name Centre of Gravity Saṅgha, and together we've explored the intersection of Yoga and Buddhism through āsana classes, prāṇāyāma courses, textual study, meditation retreats, personal meetings, and discussion. We've also benefited from wonderful guest teachers, including Norman Feldman, Richard Freeman, David Loy, Roshi Pat Enkyo O'Hara, and others.

Resisting a public face or the need to become a commercial enterprise, we've been able to quietly focus on deep practice and learn together about what works for whom and where some practices that belong to ancient Indian and Asian traditions need to be tuned by these times. That's the collective element in the inception of this book. The motivation to collect these chapters also emerges from my own quest to clarify and explore how Yoga and Buddhism work together. It is a response to the many questions from students both at Centre of Gravity and in the many other international communities in which I teach.

Elaine Jackson generously read through the first draft of my introductory chapter and in so doing helped clarify the direction of this book. Emily Bower and the family of skilled editors and designers at Shambhala Publications have again brought the dharma of type out into the world. Tessa Jones helped organize the final stages of the manuscript, Grant Hutchison helped locate artwork sources and other important details, and Heather Frise offered a perfect room for writing.

I hope this book will deepen the discussion about the intersection of these two traditions and how they might best come alive at this time, in this culture.

The contributors who have generously taken time to put their thoughts, questions, and insights into written form are all people for whom I have tremendous respect and owe a debt of gratitude. While some of the contributors I count as close friends, others I have only known through written form; nevertheless, I can intuit the growth of a larger community of thoughtful and dedicated yogins for whom the dharma of Yoga and the Buddha have had immeasurable impact.

Hopefully future yogins on the path of awakening will be inspired by this collection and take the dialogue between these traditions much further in the hope of creating a common language and set of practices that respond to the individual, collective, institutional, social, and ecological imbalances of contemporary times.

NOTES

Introduction by Michael Stone

1. Karen Armstrong, *Buddha* (New York: Penguin Putnam Inc., 2001), xxv.
2. Ibid.
3. Karen Armstrong, *A History of God* (New York: Gramercy Books, 1993), 28–29.
4. Swami Venkatesananda, *The Supreme Yoga,* vol. 1 (my own translation) (Rishikesh, India: Divine Life Society, 1976), 284–85.

Chapter 1. Awakening to Prāṇa by Chip Hartranft

1. Patañjali (author's own translation), *The Yoga Sūtra* I.2–4.
2. Ibid., II.35–39.
3. Ibid., II.40–45.
4. Ibid., II.46–48.
5. Patañjali (author's own translation), *The Yoga Sūtra* II.49–53.
6. Patañjali (author's own translation), *The Yoga Sūtra* II.54–55.
7. Ibid., III.1–3.
8. Ibid., IV.25–26.
9. Ibid., IV.29–34.
10. Author's own translation, *Majjhima Nikāya* (Oxford, Eng.: Pali Text Society, 1979), I.56.
11. Ibid.
12. Ibid.
13. Ibid.
14. Ibid.
15. Ibid.
16. Patañjali (author's own translation), *The Yoga Sūtra* II.47.
17. *Majjhima Nikāya* (Oxford, Eng.: Pali Text Society, 1979).

Chapter 2. Body and Mind Dropped Away by Roshi Pat Enkyo O'Hara

1. Norman Waddell and Masao Abe, *The Heart of Dōgen's Shobogenzo* (Albany, N.Y.: SUNY Press, 2002), 2–6.
2. The story of Dōgen's awakening is told in many places and versions. See Dōgen, *The Record of Transmitting the Light,* trans. Francis Cook (Somerville, Mass.: Wisdom Publications, 2003); and *Transmission of the Light,* trans. Thomas Cleary (San Francisco: North Point Press, 1990).
3. Carl Bielefeldt, *Dōgen's Manuals of Zen Meditation* (Berkeley, Calif.: University of California Press, 1988), 5.
4. The opening lines of poem 190 in Robert G. Henricks, *The Poetry of Han-Shan: A Complete, Annotated Translation of Cold Mountain* (Albany, N.Y.: SUNY Series in Buddhist Studies, 1990), 267.
5. This koan is translated by Thomas Yuho Kirchner in his *Entangling Vines, Zen Koans of the Shumon Kattoshu, Tenryu-Ji* (Boston: Institute for Philosophy and Religion, 2004), 13.
6. This is an old koan, found in many sources. An accessible version is in Andy Ferguson, *Zen's Chinese Heritage* (Boston: Wisdom Publications, 2000), 46.
7. Bielefeldt, *Dōgen's Manuals of Zen Meditation,* 194.
8. Kazuaki Tanahashi, trans., *Moon in a Dewdrop, Writings of Zen Master Dōgen,* by Dōgen (San Francisco: North Point Press, 1985), 85.
9. Thomas Merton, *Thoughts in Solitude* (Boston: Shambhala Publications, 1993), 103.
10. Steven Heine, *The Zen Poetry of Dōgen, "Treasury of the True Dharma-eye"* (Boston: Tuttle Publications, 1997), 103–4.
11. Burton Watson, trans. *The Vimalakirti Sūtra* (New York: Columbia University Press, 1996), 37.

Chapter 3. The Broad Tongue of the Tathāgata: Spatial Breathing in Ch'an by Ming Qing Sifu (Daniel Odier)

1. J. C. Cleary, *Zibo, the Last Great Zen Master of China* (Charlottesville, Va.: University of Virginia, 1989).
2. Xu-Yun, *Empty Cloud,* trans. Charles Luk (Rochester, Va.: Element Press, 1988), page unknown.

Chapter 4. Zen or Yoga? A Teacher Responds by Shosan Victoria Austin

1. Barbara Stoler Miller, trans., *Yoga: Discipline of Freedom,* by Patañjali (Berkeley and Los Angeles: University of California Press, 1995), x.
2. B. K. S. Iyengar, "Practice to Have Divine Grace," in *Astadala Yogamala,* vol. 3 (New Delhi: Allied Publishers Private Limited, 2002), 298.
3. Red Pine, trans., *The Zen Teaching of Bodhidharma* (San Francisco: North Point Press, 1989), 33.
4. Dōgen-zenji, *Shobogenzo Genjokoan,* unpublished translation by Victoria Austin, based on previous unpublished translations of David Chadwick, Maezumi Roshi, and Kazuaki Tanahashi, 1970.
5. Personal communication with Sojun Mel Weitsman, 2008.
6. B. K. S. Iyengar, "Yoga Defined," in *Astadala Yogamala,* vol. 1 (New Delhi: Allied Publishers Private Limited, 2000), 69.
7. Barbara Stoler Miller, *Yoga: Discipline of Freedom,* 8–9.
8. Ibid.
9. *The Bhagavad Gītā, or The Song Divine,* trans. Syt. Jayadayal Goyandaka et al. (Gorakhpur, India: Gita Press, 1997), chap. 4, verse 24.
10. Ibid. See also chap. 6, verses 16–17: "Arjuna, this Yoga is neither for him who overeats, nor for him who observes a complete fast. . . . Yoga which rids one of woe is accomplished only by him who is regulated in diet and recreation, regulated in performing actions."
11. Excerpted from San Francisco Zen Center Meal Chant.
12. "What Is a Certified Teacher of Iyengar Yoga?," *Iyengar Yoga National Association of the United States Certification Manual,* 2009 edition, s.v., chap. 1.

Chapter 5. Joining with Naturalness by Ari Goldfield and Rose Taylor

1. From *The Commentary on Valid Cognition* (Tib: tshad ma rnam 'grel; Skt: Pramana-varttika), quoted in Khenpo Tsültrim Gyamtso, blo rtags kyi rnam gzhag rigs gzhung rgya mtsho'i snying po. (New York: Nitartha International, 1997), 11. Quotation translated from Tibetan by Ari Goldfield.
2. Desire, anger, stupidity, jealousy, and arrogance.
3. From an unpublished letter by Khenpo Tsültrim Gyamtso Rinpoche, translated from Tibetan by Ari Goldfield.

4. These key points are what the authors have learned from their own teachers (primarily the Tibetan masters Chögyam Trungpa Rinpoche and Khenpo Tsültrim Gyamtso Rinpoche) and these teachers' tradition of Tibetan Buddhist practice. There are certainly a wide variety of different explanations of these terms and topics within the panorama of Buddhist traditions. Just as doctors have different medicines to give to different patients, Buddhism traditionally presents and accommodates different explanations of its views and practices. This is one of its strengths.
5. A founder of the Kagyü lineage of Tibetan Buddhism, Milarepa (1040–1123) is revered for having persevered through terrible hardship and austerity on his ultimately triumphant journey to enlightenment. His songs about his experiences and realization are renowned.
6. From Milarepa's Hundred Thousand Songs (Tib: mi la mgur 'bum), the chapter "Meeting with Paldarbum," translated by Willa Baker and Susan Skolnick, unpublished, 1997, p. 8.
7. Translated and arranged by Jim Scott ©2006.
8. The awakening mind.
9. Shantideva, *The Way of the Bodhisattva,* trans. Padmakara Translation Group (Shambhala Classics, 1997), chap. 1, verses 21–22, 34.
10. From the Tibetan text for the Kagyü lineage preliminary (ngondro) practices [Tib: sgrub brgyud rin po che'i phreng ba karma kam tshang rtogs pa'i don brgyud las byung ba'i gsung dri ma med pa rnams bkod nas ngag 'don rgyun khyer gyi rim pa 'phags lam bgrod pa'i shing rta], 9. Verse translated by Ari Goldfield.
11. Elizabeth Callahan, trans., *The King of Aspiration Prayers, the Aspiration for Noble Excellent Conduct* ©1994, verse 15.
12. Orally quoted by Khenpo Tsültrim Gyamtso Rinpoche, translated from Tibetan by Ari Goldfield.
13. Unpublished verse of Khenpo Tsültrim Gyamtso Rinpoche, translated from Tibetan by Ari Goldfield.
14. For brevity's sake, the five stages in this presentation have here been condensed into two. Books devoted to explaining all or some of these five stages in more detail include the following: Khenpo Tsültrim Gyamtso, *Progressive Stages of Meditation on Emptiness* (Oxford, Eng.: Longchen Foundation, 1986); Khenpo Tsültrim Gyamtso, *The Sun of Wisdom* (Boston: Shambhala Publications, 2003); and Khenpo Tsültrim Gyamtso, *Stars of Wisdom* (Boston: Shambhala Publications, 2010).
15. Oral teaching of Kalu Rinpoche.
16. From Milarepa's "Song of Meditating on the Generation Stage" (Tib: bskyed rim gyi gsungs mgur), translated from Tibetan by Ari Goldfield.

17. From Milarepa's "Song of the Three Nails" (Tib: gzer gsum gyi gsung mgur), translated from Tibetan by Rose Taylor ©2009.
18. Quoted in Karmapa Wangchuk Dorje's guide to Mahamudra meditation entitled *Ocean of Definitive Meaning* (Tib: phyag chen nges don rgya mtsho, Rumtek, India), Tibetan folio 104a. Translated from Tibetan by Ari Goldfield.
19. The moon's reflection on the surface of a pool of water is luminous while at the same time empty of inherent nature. In this way, it is an example of mind's true nature, the union of luminosity-emptiness.
20. Unpublished Tibetan verse by Khenpo Tsültrim Gyamtso Rinpoche, translated from Tibetan by Rose Taylor.
21. From the Tibetan version of Milarepa's *Hundred Thousand Songs, Mi la ras pa'i rnam mgur* (n.p.: mtsho sngon mi rigs dpe skrun khang, 1989), 267.
22. From Milarepa's song "The Eighteen Kinds of Yogic Joy," translated from Tibetan and arranged by Jim Scott © 1994.
23. A master of the Drukpa Kagyü lineage of Tibetan Buddhism who lived from 1189 to 1258.
24. From "The Eight Cases of Basic Goodness Not to Be Shunned," translated from Tibetan and arranged by Jim Scott © 1997.
25. Karmapa Wangchuk Dorje, *Ocean of Definitive Meaning,* Tibetan folio 121b. Verse translated by Ari Goldfield.
26. Song of Milarepa quoted in rdza dpal sprul, *kun bzang bla ma'i zhal lung* (si khron mi rigs dpe skrun khang, 1993), 538. Verse translated by Ari Goldfield.
27. "Samādhi refers to a state in which one is concentrated and not distracted. Paradoxically, it seems, the samādhi that sees everything to be like an illusion is the meditation one practices in the midst of all the distractions of thoughts and the objects that appear to the senses. When one remembers that all of these distractions are illusory, however, this constitutes the practice of this samādhi, and all the distractions are in fact friends of and enhancements to the meditation rather than hindrances or obstacles." (Khenpo Tsültrim Gyamtso, *The Sun of Wisdom* [Boston: Shambhala Publications, 2003], 53).
28. Tib: 'phags pa yang dag par sdud pa'i mdo. Quoted in Gampopa, *Jewel Ornament of Liberation* (Tib: lha rje bsod nams rin chen, dam chos yid bzhin gyi nor bu thar pa rin po che'i rgyan) (Electronic edition, Kathmandu: Pema Karpo Translation Committee, 179). Verse translated from Tibetan by Ari Goldfield.
29. Unpublished verse by Khenpo Tsültrim Gyamtso Rinpoche, translated from Tibetan by Ari Goldfield.
30. Chögyam Trungpa, *The Collected Works of Chögyam Trungpa,* vol. 7 (Boston: Shambhala Publications, 2004), 47.

Chapter 6. Zen Body by Eido Shimano Roshi

1. My translation.

Chapter 8. Brahmā Vihāra, Emptiness, and Ethics by Christopher Key Chapple

1. The full verse reads:
   maitrīkaruṇāmudita upekṣā
   sukha duḥkha puṇya apunyam
   visayanam bhavanatasca citta prasadanam (*Yoga Sūtra* [*YS*] I.33)
2. The nine types are given as follows: (1) Reformer, (2) Helper, (3) Motivator, (4) Artist, (5) Thinker, (6) Loyalist, (7) Generalist, (8) Leader, (9) Peacemaker. See Don Richard Riso, *Understanding the Enneagram: The Practical Guide to Personality Types* (Boston: Houghton Mifflin, 1990), 35–88.
3. See the chapter titled "The Feminine Gender in Patañjali's Description of Yogic Practices" in Chapple, *Yoga and the Luminous: Patañjali's Spiritual Path to Freedom* (Albany, N.Y.: SUNY Press, 2008), 237–48.
4. Haribhadra's *Yogadrstisamuccaya* correlates eight goddesses to the eight limbs of Yoga: Mitra/yama; Tārā/niyāma; Bala/āsana; Dipra/prāṇāyāma; Shtira/pratyāhāra; Kanta/dhāraṇā; Prabha/dhyāna; Para/samādhi. See Christopher Key Chapple, *Reconciling Yogas: Haribhadra's Collection of Views on Yoga* (Albany, N.Y.: SUNY Press, 2003), 20.
5. Philip Kapleau, *The Wheel of Death* (New York: Harper, 1971), 82–83. Efforts were made to obtain more information about this translation but none was available.
6. Christopher Chapple, *The Yoga Sūtras of Patañjali: An Analysis of the Sanskrit with Accompanying English Translation* (Delhi, India: Sri Satguru Publications, 1990), *YS* I.43.
7. Ibid., *YS* III.3.
8. Ibid., *YS* IV.34.
9. Ibid., *YS* IV.21.
10. Ibid., *YS* II.35–39.
11. Chapple, *Yoga and the Luminous State*, *YS* I.48.
12. Chapple, *The Yoga Sūtras of Patañjali*, *YS* I.39.

13. For an account of this training, see "Rāja Yoga and the Guru: Gurani Anjali of Yoga Anand Ashram, Amityville, New York," in *Gurus in America,* ed. Thomas A. Forshtoefel and Cynthia Ann Humes (Albany, N.Y.: SUNY Press, 2005), 15–34.
14. Chapple, *Yoga and the Luminous State.* See the chapter "Precepts and Vows in Yoga and Jainism," 31–48, for various narrative examples.
15. Har Dayal, *The Bodhisattva Doctrine in Buddhist Sanskrit Literature* (New York: Samuel Weiser, 1932), 291.
16. Vijnanabhiksu, *Yogasarasangraha* (Madras, India: Theosophical Press, 1933), 17.

Chapter 9. Buddha and the Yogi: Paradigms of Restraint and Renunciation by Mu Soeng

1. For an overview of the culture of Yoga at the time of the Buddha, see Sukumar Dutt, *Buddhist Monks and Monasteries of India: Their History and Their Contribution to Indian Culture* (Ann Arbor: Univ. of Michigan Press, 1962, 2009), especially pp. 35–52. Also see A. K. Warder, *Indian Buddhism* (Delhi, India: Motilal Bonarsidass, 1970), 27–41. Another overview of the era's religious practices is provided in A. L. Basham, *The Wonder That Was India* (London: Sidgwick and Jackson, 1987), 232–345. See also Winston L. King, "Theravāda Meditation: The Buddhist Transformation of Yoga" (Charlottesville, Va.: Univ. of Virginia Press, 1980), 1–17.
2. For an overview of ascetic practices in contemporary Hinduism in India see Sondra L. Hausner, *Wandering with Sādhus: Ascetics in the Hindu Himalayas* (Bloomington: Indiana Univ. Press, 2007). Also of interest is Dolf Hartsuiker, *Sādhus: Holy Men of India* (Rochester, Vt.: Inner Traditions, 1993). For a more personal account of these practices half a century ago, see Agehananda Bharati, *The Tantric Tradition* (London: Rider Press, 1966). These are only three of numerous other accounts, both personal and anthropological, of the continuation of ascetic practices among yogis in India.
3. Joseph P. Amar, "On Hermits and Desert Dwellers," in *Ascetic Behavior in Greco-Roman Antinquity: A Sourcebook,* ed. Vincent L. Wimbush. See also Owen Chadwick, *Western Asceticism,* on the background of asceticism within early Christianity.
4. Middle-Length Discourses of the Buddha (*Majjhima Nikāya*), suttas 5.29 and 32.7; these ascetic practices are mentioned in various places in the Pali texts, but never together in the same place.

Chapter 10. A Twisted Story by Jill Satterfield

1. Thanissaro Bhikkhu, *Satipaṭṭhānā Sutta,* MN10 (www.accesstoinsight.org).
2. B. K. S. Iyengar, *Light on Yoga* (New York: Schocken Books, 1966), 28.
3. T. K. V. Desikachar, *The Heart of Yoga: Developing a Personal Practice* (Rochester, Vt.: Inner Traditions International, 1995), 155.
4. Kalu Rinpoche, *The Gem Ornament of Manifold Instructions,* ed. Caroline M. Parke and Nancy J. Clarke (Ithaca, N.Y.: Snow Lion Publications, 1987).
5. Bokar Rinpoche and Khenpo Donyo, *The Profound Wisdom of the Heart Sūtra* (Ashland, Ohio: Clear Point Press, 1994).
6. Tulku Thondup, *Enlightened Journey: Buddhist Practice as Everyday Life* (Boston: Shambhala Publications, 1995).

Chapter 11. Mindfulness Yoga by Frank Jude Boccio

1. Georg Feuerstein, *The Yoga Tradition: Its History, Literature, Philosophy and Practice* (Prescott, Ariz.: Hohm Press, 1998), 7.
2. Bhikkhu Bodhi, *The Connected Discourses of the Buddha: A Translation of the Samyutta Nikāya* (Somerville, Mass.: Wisdom Publications, 2000), 157–58.
3. Georg Feuerstein, trans., *The Yoga-Sūtra of Patañjali: A New Translation and Commentary* (Rochester, Vt.: Inner Traditions, 1989), book 2, verses 46 and 47.
4. Chip Hartranft, trans., *The Yoga-Sūtra of Patañjali: A New Translation with Commentary* (Boston: Shambhala Publications, 2003), book 2, verses 46 and 47.
5. Ibid., book 2, verse 48.
6. Bhikkhu Nanamoli, *The Life of the Buddha* (Kandy, Sri Lanka: Buddhist Publication Society, 1992), 14.
7. Ibid.
8. Thich Nhat Hanh, *Our Appointment with Life: The Buddha's Teaching on Living in the Present* (Berkeley, Calif.: Parallax Press, 1990), 5.
9. Hartranft, *The Yoga-Sūtra of Patañjali,* book 1, verse 1.
10. Frank Jude Boccio, *Mindfulness Yoga: The Awakened Union of Breath, Body and Mind* (Somerville, Mass.: Wisdom Publications, 2004), 47.
11. Ibid., 188, translation by the author.
12. *Genjo Koan,* freely translated and adapted by the author.

Chapter 12. The Body of Truth by Ajahn Amaro Bhikkhu

1. *Majjhima Nikāya,* sutta 43, "The Greater Series of Questions and Answers," par. 9, author's own rendering.
2. Ibid., sutta 119, "The Discourse on Mindfulness of the Body," par. 22, author's own rendering.
3. *Samyutta Nikāya,* section 43 of the Connected Discourses, "Mindfulness Directed Toward the Body," sutta 1, par. 3, author's own rendering.
4. *Majjhima Nikāya,* sutta 10, "The Discourse on the Foundations of Mindfulness," par. 2–3, author's own rendering. And *Dīgha Nikāya,* sutta 22, "The Greater Discourse on the Foundations of Mindfulness," par. 1, author's own rendering.
5. This passage can be found in a number of places in the scriptures, often when the Buddha is being offered a place to establish a monastery; for example, he said this when the generous donor Anathapindika was inspired to provide such a place, as mentioned at *Cullavagga* 6.4, in the books of monastic discipline. This lay supporter then purchased Prince Jeta's Grove, as legend has it, by covering the ground with gold coins.
6. Ajahn Chah, *Food for the Heart* (Somerville, Mass.: Wisdom Publications, 2002), 371–72.
7. Ajahn Amaro, traditional oral teaching, 2009.
8. *Dhammapada,* verse 1, lines 3–4, author's own rendering.
9. Joseph Campbell, *Oriental Mythology, Brihadarañayaka Upanishad* 1.4.1–5 (New York: Viking Penguin, 1962), 14.
10. Jill Satterfield, personal communication, 2008.
11. Ibid.
12. Richard B. Clarke, *Verses on the Faith-Mind* (Buffalo, N.Y.: White Pine Press, 2001), 3.
13. Jill Satterfield, personal communication, 2008.
14. Mary Pafford, personal communication, 2008.

Chapter 13. Practice Maps of the Great Yogis by Michael Stone

1. Personal communication during teachings of Yoga Vasiṣta with Pandit Upadya at Hindu Temple, Fern Ave., Toronto. Author's translation.
2. Dōgen, quoted in Robert Aitken, *Mind of Clover* (New York: North Point Press, 1984), 119.
3. *Dhammapada* (author's own translation), lines 153–54.

4. *Rig Veda,* trans. Wendy Doniger (London: Penguin, 1981), 2.16.
5. *Kalama Sutta,* trans. Soma Thera, *The Wheel* no. 8 (Kandy, Sri Lanka: Buddhist Publication Society, 1987), 32.
6. *Canki Sutta, The Middle-Length Discourses of the Buddha,* trans. Bhikku Nanamoli and Bhikku Bodhi (Somerville, Mass.: Wisdom Publications, 1995), sutta 95, par. 14–25.
7. Stephen Batchelor, *Verses from the Center* (New York: Riverhead Books, 2000), 116.
8. Don Cupitt, *Emptiness and Brightness* (Santa Rosa, Calif.: Polebridge Press, 2001), 22.
9. John Daido Loori, *Invoking Reality: Moral and Ethical Teachings of Zen* (Boston: Shambhala Publications, 2007), 33.
10. There is no clear or final demarcation between Indian systems of thought, especially since most schools of Indian philosophy grew out of one another. Systems of Indian philosophy, whether Buddhist, Hindu, or Jain, as examples, have always been debating with one another, even in the time of the Buddha, and thus it is unrealistic to expect that the lines that define one tradition from another be absolute or obvious. In fact, it's often cited that there are six main schools of Indian philosophy, but "this view is problematic," writes philosopher Richard King, "firstly because it is a mistake to impose the idea of 'orthodoxy' onto Indian religion and culture. Even when discussing philosophical perspectives it is clear that there has never been a centralizing institution comparable to the Christian Church to oversee and define doctrinal correctness within India."

    Of the six primary schools of "orthodox Indian philosophy" (Nyāya, Vaisesika, Sāṃkyha, Yoga, Mimāṃsā, Vedānta), not one includes Buddhism, and in fact, when one looks deeply into the varied forms of Indian philosophy, we see that the schools classified as the six main schools change at different times. Although this may be frustrating and peculiar for the academic or logician, it reminds the practitioner just how fluid the systems really are.
11. Red Pine, trans., *The Heart Sūtra,* line 19 (Washington, D.C.: Shoemaker & Hoard, 2004), 3.
12. Thanissaro Bhikkhu, trans., *Satipathana Sutta: Frames of Reference* 1.1 (2009), www.accesstoinsight.org/tipitaka/mn/mn.010.than.html.
13. Case 20, *The Book of Serenity,* trans. Thomas Cleary (Boston: Shambhala Publications, 2003).
14. Chip Hartranft, trans., *Yoga-Sūtra of Patañjali* (Boston: Shambhala Publications, 2003), 104.
15. Seng-ts'an, "Relying on Mind," in *The Roaring Stream,* ed. Nelson Foster and Jack Shoemaker (New York: The Ecco Press, 1996), 12.
16. *Netra Tantra* 8.11, quoted in Swami Lakshmanjoo, *Self Realization in Kashmir Shaivism,* ed. John Hughes (Albany, N.Y.: SUNY Press, 1998), 84.

17. Reginald Ray, *Touching Enlightenment: Finding Realization in the Body* (Boulder, Colo.: SoundsTrue, 2008), xl.
18. Takuan, *The Mysterious Record of Immovable Wisdom,* quoted in Foster and Shoemaker, eds., *The Roaring Stream,* 277.
19. *Hatha Yoga Pradīpikā* attributed to Svātmarama, chap. 4, line 113. My own translation based on previous translation by Pancham Sinh, *The Hatha Yoga Pradīpikā* (New Delhi: Munshiram Manoharlal Publishers, Ltd., 1914–15).
20. Chip Hartranft, *The Yoga-Sūtra of Patañjali,* 80.
21. Ibid., 80–81.
22. The outlook is described in a classic story from the *Chandogya Upaniṣad.* Uddālaka, the father of Shwetaketu, starts explaining to his son about ParaBrahmā Tattva and says, "It is not amenable to any kind of testimony. It cannot be perceived through sense organs. Even the mind cannot reach it." Shwetaketu finds it difficult to believe his father's words. "If Brahmā were to pervade the entire creation, why is it that it cannot be perceived by the sense organs?" he argues. While the conversation proceeds, it is getting dark. Continuing to instruct his son about ParaBrahmā, Uddālaka asks him to bring a big pot of water and to place two big pieces of rock salt in it. Shwetaketu does exactly as his father tells him. He can now see, illuminated by the light of the stars and the moon, the two lumps of salt in the water. Uddālaka asks his son to cover the pot with a plate. He says that he will continue the following morning and tells his son to go to bed. The next day, after the morning rituals, the father asks his son to take out the lumps of salt. Shwetaketu removes the lid of the pot and finds that the pieces of salt are not there! He puts his hand inside and searches thoroughly. He can find nothing. He father smiles and says, "Put a few drops of that water into your mouth." Shwetaketu allows a few drops of the water to drop on his tongue and says, "Gee! It is salty." Now Uddālaka asks his son to taste the water from different parts of that pot. Regardless of where it is taken from, the water is equally salty. "What did you learn from this?" asks the father. Shwetaketu says, "I understand that the lumps of salt that I put in to this water pot have dissolved and have equally spread in this water." Uddālaka says, "See! The salt is present everywhere in this pot of water. Still, your eyes or your fingers cannot perceive it! Only your tongue is able to perceive. Similarly, the Ātma pervades the body, the Indriyas, and so on. Still, no sense organ can perceive it! We can perceive this fundamental spiritual reality only through inference."
23. Joan Halifax, oral teaching and personal communication, Upaya Zen Center, Santa Fe, 2007.
24. Robert Bringhurst, *Everywhere Being Is Dancing* (Halifax, Nova Scotia: Gaspereau Press, 2007), page unknown.
25. Reb Anderson, *Warm Smiles from Cold Mountains* (Berkeley, Calif.: Rodmell Press, 2005), 118.

CONTRIBUTOR BIOGRAPHIES

VEN. AMARO BHIKKHU, born in England in 1956, received his BSc. in Psychology and Physiology from the University of London. Spiritual searching led him to Thailand, where he went to Wat Pah Nanachat, a Forest Tradition monastery established for Western disciples of Thai meditation master Ajahn Chah, who ordained him as a bhikkhu in 1979. He returned to England and joined Ajahn Sumedho at the newly established Chithurst Monastery. He resided for many years at the Amaravati Buddhist Centre north of London, making trips to California every year during the 1990s. Since June 1996 he has lived at Abhayagiri Monastery. He has written an account of his 830-mile trek from Chithurst to Harnham Vihāra called *Tudong—the Long Road North,* republished in the expanded book *Silent Rain,* and he published another book, *Small Boat, Great Mountain—Theravādan Reflections on the Natural Great Perfection,* in 2003. On June 16, 2005, Ajahn Amaro returned to Abhayagiri after spending one year on sabbatical visiting Buddhist holy places in India, Nepal, and Bhutan.

SHOSAN VICTORIA AUSTIN was ordained as a Soto Zen priest in 1982, started teaching Iyengar Yoga in 1984, and has taught continuously in both traditions for many years. She studies Yoga with Manouso Manos in San Francisco and with the Iyengars in India. Victoria currently serves as a Dharma Teacher-at-Large at San Francisco Zen Center and as a Nito-kyoshi of the Sotoshu. She teaches at the Abode of Iyengar Yoga, the Iyengar Yoga Institute of San Francisco Teacher Training Program, and varied settings including hospitals, workplaces, and meditation centers.

Poep Sa Frank Jude Boccio, a certified Yoga teacher and ordained Zen Buddhist teacher, is also an Interfaith minister, and a lay brother in the Tiep Hien Order established by Thich Nhat Hanh. His eclectic approach is influenced by his study of a variety of Yoga approaches as well as his many years of dharma practice, evidenced by his emphasis on mindfulness and compassionate action (karuṇā). He has written for *Yoga Journal*, *Tricycle*, *Shambhala Sun*, and other journals. His book, *Mindfulness Yoga: The Awakened Union of Breath, Body, and Mind*, is the only full-length treatment applying the Buddha's mindfulness meditation teachings on the Four Establishments of Mindfulness to Yoga āsana practice. He lives in Tucson, Arizona, with his wife, Monica, and their two cats, Sula and Gotami. He travels wherever he is invited, throughout the world, offering workshops, trainings, and retreats. For further information he can be contacted through www.mindfulnessyoga.net.

Christopher Key Chapple is Doshi Professor of Indic and Comparative Theology at Loyola Marymount University in Los Angeles, where he has taught since 1985. A specialist in the religions of India, he has published more than a dozen books, including *Yoga and the Luminous: Patañjali's Spiritual Path to Freedom*. He is the editor of the journal *Worldviews: Global Religions, Culture, and Ecology* (Brill) and serves on numerous advisory boards. He won the Rajinder and Jyoti Gandhi Book Award for Excellence in Dharma Studies in 2008. He and his wife, Maureen, trained in meditative Yoga for twelve years under the guidance of Gurani Añjali at Yoga Anand Ashram in Amityville, New York. In 2002 he established a series of Extension training programs in Yoga and Buddhist Studies at LMU, and in 2004 established the Hill Street Center, a meditation cooperative in Santa Monica.

EIDO SHIMANO ROSHI, born in Tokyo in 1932, has been living and teaching in America for over forty years. He trained at Ryutaku-ji Monastery in Mishima, Japan, under Soen Nakagawa Roshi, from whom he received dharma transmission in 1972. Today he serves as the abbot and spiritual teacher of two practice centers in the Japanese Rinzai Zen tradition: New York Zendo Shobo-ji, on the Upper East Side of Manhattan, and Dai Bosatsu Zendo Kongo-ji, deep in the Catskill Mountains of upstate New York. He also travels regularly to Japan and Europe, where he conducts retreats and seminars.

ARI GOLDFIELD is a Buddhist translator and teacher who has studied and practiced under the close guidance of Khenpo Tsültrim Gyamtso Rinpoche since 1995. He has translated and cotranslated books, articles, texts, and numerous songs of realization on Buddhist philosophy and meditation, including Khenpo Rinpoche's "Song of the Eight Flashing Lances" teaching, which appeared in *The Best Buddhist Writing 2007*, as well as Rinpoche's books *The Sun of Wisdom* and *Stars of Wisdom*. He studied Buddhist texts in Tibetan and Sanskrit at Buddhist monasteries in Nepal and India, and at the Central Institute for Higher Tibetan Studies in India. Since 1998, he has served Rinpoche full time as secretary and translator, accompanying him on seven round-the-world teaching tours. In 2006, Rinpoche stayed in retreat and sent Ari on his own tour to teach philosophy, meditation, and yogic exercise and dance in Europe, North America, and Asia. In 2007, Rinpoche named him president of the Marpa Foundation, a nonprofit that operates under Rinpoche's direction and supports a variety of dharma activities. He holds a BA from Harvard College and a JD from Harvard Law School, both with honors.

CHIP HARTRANFT, PT, bridges the traditions of Yoga and Buddhism. He is the founding director of the Arlington Center, dedicated to the integration of Yoga and dharma practice, and has taught a blend of Yoga movement and mindfulness meditation in the Boston area since 1978. He is the author of *The Yoga-Sūtra of Patañjali: A New Translation with Commentary* and the forthcoming *How the Buddha Taught Meditation.* Chip teaches Yoga and dharma at teacher trainings and retreats across the country, including the Mindfulness Yoga and Meditation Training at Spirit Rock, and leads a week-long retreat, "The Yoga of Awakening," every February at Pura Vida in Costa Rica.

CH'AN MASTER MING QING (DANIEL ODIER) is a disciple of Ch'an master Jing Hui from the Bailin Monastery, China, where Zhaozhou lived and taught. Master Jing Hui is the successor of the great Xu Yun (Empty Cloud). Ming Qing is the author of *Ch'an and Zen, the Garden of the Iconoclasts.*

MU SOENG, a former Zen monk and teacher, is the resident scholar at the Barre Center for Buddhist Studies. He is the author of *Thousand Peaks: Korean Zen–Tradition and Teachers; Heart Sūtra: Ancient Buddhist Wisdom in the Light of Quantum Reality; Diamond Sūtra: Transforming the Way We Perceive the World;* and *Trust in Mind: The Rebellion of Chinese Zen*. He lives in Barre, Massachusetts.

ROSHI PAT ENKYO O'HARA, PHD, is the abbot of the Village Zendo. A Soto Zen Priest and certified Zen teacher, she received dharma transmission in both the Soto and Rinzai lines of Zen Buddhism, through the White Plum Lineage. Roshi currently serves as the Guiding Spiritual Teacher for the New York Center for Contemplative Care. She also serves as Co–Spiritual Director of the Zen Peacemaker Family, a spiritual, study, and social action association. Enkyo Roshi's focus is on the expression of Zen through caring, service, and creative response. Her "Five Expressions of Zen" form the matrix of study at the Village Zendo: meditation, study, communication, action, and caring.

SARAH POWERS began teaching in 1987. She interweaves the insights and practices of Yoga and Buddhism into an integral practice to enliven the body, heart, and mind. Her Yoga style blends both a Yin sequence of floor poses to enhance the meridian and organ systems, combined with a flow or Yang practice, influenced by ViniYoga, Ashtanga, and Iyengar teachings. Sarah feels that enlivening the physical and pranic bodies, as well as learning to open to our emotional difficulties, is paramount for preparing one to deepen and nourish insights into one's essential nature—a natural state of awareness. She draws from her studies in Transpersonal Psychology, as well as her in-depth training in the Vipassana, tantric, and Dzogchen practices of Buddhism. Sarah and her husband, Ty Powers, live in the San Francisco Bay Area and have created the Insight Yoga Institute (www.insightyogainstitute.com), which offers five-hundred-hour trainings with other renowned teachers blending Yoga, Buddhism, and psychology. She is cofounder of Metta Journeys (www.mettajourneys.com), a service-oriented organization that offers Yoga retreats internationally to help women and children in developing countries. Sarah is also the author of the book *Insight Yoga*. To learn more about her, see her DVDs *Insight Yoga* and *Yin and Vinyasa*, or go to www.sarahpowers.com.

JILL SATTERFIELD is the founder of Vajra Yoga and Meditation, an intuitive synthesis of Yoga and Buddhism that combines meditation, Yoga āsanas, and visualization practices. An artist by nature and training, Jill turned to Yoga thirty years ago in an effort to heal from a debilitating physical condition coupled with acute chronic pain. She has been practicing ever since and has been teaching for the past twenty years. In 1992, she began to extend her exploration of the integral relationship of the mind and body through the study of Buddhism. Through combining the two disciplines—Yoga and Buddhism—she healed beyond her own expectations and all medical prognoses, and in the process discovered her life's work. For the past sixteen years, Jill has been traveling and teaching Vajra Yoga with some of the most respected Buddhist teachers of our time. Jill is on the faculty of Spirit Rock Meditation Center's Mindfulness Training for Yoga Teachers, Kripalu Institute's Integrative Leadership Program, and is the founder of the Social Action Teacher Training—a not-for-profit developed as a professional Yoga and meditation training for teaching at-risk youth and adults, people living in chronic pain and illness, and those in recovery programs. For further information, go to www.vajrayoga.com.

MICHAEL STONE is a Yoga teacher, author, and psychotherapist and leads Centre of Gravity Saṅgha in Toronto, a diverse community of Yoga and Buddhist practitioners interested in the intersection of committed practice, social action, and daily urban life. Michael's interest revolves around integrating traditional Yoga practices in the context of community, where independent study and critical inquiry are encouraged. He teaches Yoga, meditation, and psychology in academic and clinical settings internationally, and his Yoga retreats integrate Yoga posture practice, meditation, and textual study. He is the author of *The Inner Tradition of Yoga* and *Yoga for a World Out of Balance.* For further information, visit www.centreofgravity.org.

ROSE TAYLOR is a Buddhist translator of Tibetan, second-generation Buddhist teacher, and longtime Yoga practitioner. She served as editor of *Yoga in the Rockies* and *Elephant* magazines, and has taught Buddhist meditation, philosophy, yogic exercise and dance, and classical Tibetan language to Westerners, as well as to the nuns at her teacher Khenpo Tsültrim Gyamtso Rinpoche's nunneries in Bhutan and Nepal. She is the cotranslator of Rinpoche's book *Stars of Wisdom,* and has translated numerous prayers and songs of realization. She holds an MA in Indo-Tibetan Buddhist studies from Naropa University. Having studied and practiced extensively in the Shambhala lineage, in which her mother is also a longtime student and teacher, she began training under Khenpo Rinpoche's close guidance in 2002. She currently works on translation and as an officer and administrator of Marpa Foundation.

ROBERT THURMAN is Professor of Indo-Tibetan Buddhist Studies in the Department of Religion at Columbia University, President of Tibet House, U.S., a nonprofit organization dedicated to the preservation and promotion of Tibetan civilization, and President of the American Institute of Buddhist Studies. The first American to have been ordained a Tibetan Buddhist monk and a personal friend of the Dalai Lama for over forty years, Professor Thurman is a passionate advocate and spokesperson for the truth regarding the current Tibet-China situation and the human rights violations suffered by the Tibetan people under Chinese rule. His commitment to finding a peaceful, win-win solution for Tibet and China inspired him to write his latest book, *Why the Dalai Lama Matters: His Act of Truth as the Solution for China, Tibet and the World*, published in June 2008. Thurman's work and insights are grounded in more than thirty-five years of serious academic scholarship. He has BA, AM, and PhD degrees from Harvard and has studied in Tibetan Buddhist monasteries in India and the United States.

CONTRIBUTOR CREDITS

ILLUSTRATION CREDITS

Page 211: Drawings of Yoga asana, Kathmandu, Nepal, circa nineteenth century. Reproduced with permission from Lokesh Chandra, *Dictionary of Buddhist Iconography,* vol. 1 (New Delhi: International Academy of Indian Culture and Aditya Prakashan, 1999), 94–99.

Page 214: Cosmic form of Viṣṇu-Kṛṣna with cakras originally photographed in Rajasthan, India, nineteenth century. Photographer unknown. Gouache on paper. Reproduced in Philip Rawson, *The Art of Tantra* (London: Thames and Hudson, 1973), 159.

Page 216: From a set of six paintings of the meditations on the cakras, once forming a continuous scroll depicting emptiness. Rajasthan, India, nineteenth century. Photograph by Jeff Teasedale, reproduced in Philip Rawson, *The Art of Tantra* (London: Thames and Hudson, 1973), 167.

Page 217: Image of Moolādhara cakra reproduced with permission from Swami Satyadharma, *Yoga Chudamani Upanishad* (Bihar: Yoga Publications Trust, 2003), 40.

Page 219: Illustrations from *Eighty-four Siddhas in the Jodhpur Tradition,* originally found in the Jogapradīpiakā, a text that is preserved in the British Library, London. Reproduced with permission in Gudrutn Buhnemann, *Eighty-four Āsanas in Yoga* (New Delhi: D. K. Printworld, 2007), 70.

Page 222: Diagram of the six cakras in the subtle body, Himachal Pradesh, India, eighteenth century. Reproduced in Philip Rawson, *The Art of Tantra* (London: Thames and Hudson, 1973), 162.